Heal Your
Leaky Gut

Heal Your Leaky Gut

The Hidden Cause of Many Chronic Diseases

David Brownstein, MD
with
Jodie Gould

Humanix Books

Heal Your Leaky Gut
Copyright © 2017 by Humanix Books
All rights reserved

Humanix Books, P.O. Box 20989, West Palm Beach, FL 33416, USA
www.humanixbooks.com | info@humanixbooks.com

Library of Congress Control Number: 2017938659

Cover Design: Design by Tom Lau
Interior Design: Scribe Inc.

Humanix Books is a division of Humanix Publishing, LLC. Its trademark,
consisting of the word "Humanix," is registered in the Patent and Trademark
Office and in other countries.

Disclaimer: The information presented in this book is meant to be used for
general resource purposes only; it is not intended as specific medical advice
for any individual and should not substitute medical advice from a health care
professional. If you have (or think you may have) a medical problem, speak to
your doctor or health care practitioner immediately about your risk and possible
treatments. Do not engage in any therapy or treatment without consulting a
medical professional.

ISBN: 978-1-63006-080-0 (Hardcover)
ISBN: 978-1-63006-081-7 (E-book)

Printed in the United States of America
10 9 8 7 6 5 4 3 2

Contents

Introduction

Angela, a thirty-three-year-old registered nurse, came to me with stomach pains, which she had been having for a year. It started after a particularly stressful event in her life, from which she never recovered. Since that time, she suffered from bouts of diarrhea, constipation, and bloating. The only time of the day she felt good was in the morning before eating. As soon as food hit her stomach, the pain would start. She saw three different doctors, all of whom diagnosed her with irritable bowel syndrome (IBS). They gave her different medications, none of which worked. Not one of the doctors talked to her about her diet, even though she asked them if her IBS (a.k.a. leaky gut) was caused by something she ate. One of the doctors, a gastroenterologist, told her, "It doesn't matter what you eat."

She came to me frustrated that she wasn't getting better and asked if there were any alternative treatments that could help. I gave her a physical exam and took a complete medical and dietary history. I discovered that Angela's diet was loaded with dairy, including lots of cheese, and refined carbohydrates such as bread and pasta. When I asked if any particular foods bothered her, she said, "All foods bother me." Her stomach was tender, and even a light touch would make her moan in pain.

Her lab tests revealed that she had a high level of antibodies in her system (large *Y*-shaped proteins recruited by the immune system to identify and neutralize foreign objects like bacteria and viruses) from cow's milk protein called casein. This did not surprise me because the majority of the people I see are allergic to casein. She also tested positive for *H. pylori*, a bacterial infection of the stomach lining that 70 percent of people have without realizing it because they have no symptoms. I treated her with an herbal therapy consisting of oregano oil, Citricidal (made from grapefruit rind), and mastic, an herb from the Mediterranean that peer-reviewed studies have shown works with nearly 100 percent efficacy in treating *H. pylori*. I told Angela to adopt a dairy-free diet. When I saw her again eight weeks later, she was fully recovered.

I see patients like Angela with painful, leaky guts all the time. They come in sick of feeling sick and looking for something (anything) that will make them feel better and enjoy food (and life) again. If they are taking medications, and most are, they are suffering from the side effects of the drugs that are supposed to heal them. I used to be one of those doctors who prescribed whatever "approved" drugs were thought to treat the problem at hand. That was before I learned that using drugs and expecting them to improve the long-term function of your body is like putting water or orange juice instead of motor oil into your car's engine and expecting it to run smoothly.

My Story

All I've ever wanted for as long as I can remember is to be a family doctor. I came from a traditional household where we went to doctors when we were sick and did whatever they said. In my family, we never thought to question our physicians. So when I went to college at the University of Michigan, I took the traditional, requisite premed courses and received my medical degree from Wayne State University in Detroit. Again, I never questioned what I was taught in medical school.

I remember taking one three-hour course in nutrition—that was it. I did not think much of that class, as nutrition was not emphasized in my medical training. I did become an expert in diagnosing illnesses and prescribing the right medication to treat those illnesses. (I didn't know then that much of what I was taught in medical school was incorrect.) I vividly remember telling my patients not to take supplements because they would be wasting their money. My mother-in-law, who was a big believer in nutrition and supplements, used to give me articles about both, but I was steadfast in my conviction that there was no science behind any of it. (Trust me, as I began to embrace the use of nutraceuticals, she never failed to remind me of my initial doubt.)

I did my residency at a busy family practice in Michigan and then began my own practice in a suburb of Detroit, where I was about to become a partner. Six months in, however, I started losing sleep, and I couldn't figure out why. After many sleepless nights, I woke up one day and told my wife, "I don't want to be a doctor anymore!" I was twenty-nine years old, I was $90,000 in debt from student loans, and my wife was pregnant with our first child. "What are you talking about?"

she asked incredulously. (There were a few other words said here, but that is between her and me.)

"I just don't like how I am practicing medicine," I said. "All I'm doing is treating people with drugs that aren't really working and then having to use more medication to treat the side effects. I'm not really helping anybody," I told her. "I can't see myself doing this for the next thirty or forty years." My wife suggested I do another residency, but that would just be more of the same. She could see how painfully unhappy I was, but we were at a loss for what I should do next.

Around this time, a friend encouraged me to meet with a local chiropractor named Dr. Robert Radtke. I was reluctant to see him because, at that time, I used to advise my patients to stay away from chiropractors. However, due to my lack of sleep and my anxiety, I set up a meeting for the following week. When the meeting day came, I told my wife I was going to cancel, as I felt it would be a waste of my time. After all, why did I need to meet with a chiropractor when I didn't even believe in them? She said that would be rude and told me to go see him and "be nice."

As it turned out, Dr. Radtke was a very smart doctor. He knew a tremendous amount about nutrition, which I didn't know about, and he talked about treating patients with vitamins, minerals, herbs, and the chiropractic philosophy. He was schooled on entirely different therapies than I was. In fact, I knew little to nothing about the therapies he was having success with. Dr. Radtke gave me a book called *Healing with Nutrition* by Jonathan Wright, MD, an allopathic practitioner. I read it cover to cover late into the night.

After that, I decided to learn as much as I could about holistic medicine. That was twenty-four years ago, and there wasn't as much information on the subject as there is today. I had to essentially retrain myself. I went back to my biochemistry books and studied the mechanism of action of the drugs I was indoctrinated to use. What I learned shocked me. I learned that most drugs don't support the body's biochemistry and physiology; they inhibit it, because drugs work by poisoning the enzymes and blocking the receptors in the body. I wrote about this in my book *Drugs That Don't Work and Natural Therapies That Do!* Unfortunately, medical schools don't teach us how to enhance the body's biochemical pathways—we're taught how to block it.

After discovering this new and, to me, revelatory way to treat patients, I decided to leave my practice to work as a family doctor at the Detroit Medical Center. I told my new employer that I wanted to practice holistic medicine, and they didn't know what that was, but they were in agreement. At this office, I immediately called my first patient—my dad, who had been sick for years—and asked him to come in so I could do bloodwork. My father had his first heart attack at forty and his second at forty-two. Over the intervening twenty years, he had two bypass surgeries and numerous angioplasties, and he was on twelve different medications for diabetes, blood pressure, angina, and cholesterol. Due to my studying of holistic principles, I initially tested my father's thyroid and testosterone levels, which the best doctors in town had never checked. The results showed that his testosterone was below detectable limits, and his thyroid hormone levels were near the bottom of the acceptable range.

I immediately put my dad on natural thyroid hormones and natural testosterone. Within a few days, his face changed from pale and pasty to a healthier pink. After seven days, the angina that had plagued him for twenty years went away and never returned. A month later, his low-density lipoprotein (LDL; the "bad" cholesterol), which had been stuck at 300 mg/dl (190 mg/dl is considered very high), dropped to

200 mg/dl without even changing his bad diet or exercising. When I saw those changes occur in my dad, I knew I was on the right path and that I could finally heal people. Since that moment, I have not stopped reading, studying, and going to meetings to learn more about how best to support the body's ability to maintain optimal health.

I continued to practice holistic medicine for the next five years before becoming a faculty member at Wayne State. Wayne State operated one of the first holistic practices in the country associated with a medical school. In 1998 (with my partners, doctors Ng and Nusbaum), I founded the Center for Holistic Medicine in West Bloomfield, Michigan, where I am currently medical director. I've treated thousands of patients, and I've written fourteen self-published health books that have sold more than half a million copies.

What Is Leaky Gut Syndrome?

Leaky gut syndrome (LGS) occurs when the lining of the small intestine is damaged, allowing foreign compounds to escape into your bloodstream, which weakens your immune system and triggers autoimmune reactions. There are so many myths and misconceptions about how to best support the gut, many of which come from gastroenterologists, who deal with plumbing problems but know nothing about the functional aspects of the gut.

Here's how it works. Your gut is directly related to the health of your whole body. We are designed to absorb nutrients that support our bodies and help us make energy and get rid of things that we don't need or are toxic. Gut cells are lined together like bricks. There are little openings that allow nutrients to be absorbed and help the bad stuff pass through to be excreted. When you have a "leaky gut," those bricks have spaces between them, and they get broken down so everything is absorbed, including the bad stuff. When this happens, you get inflammation, and the immune system is compromised.

I decided to write about LGS after finding that many of my patients' illnesses, from arthritis, IBS, acid reflux, diarrhea, and constipation to chronic fatigue, fibromyalgia, and autoimmune diseases, are caused by this strange-sounding condition. Similarly, if you have depression, muscle and joint pain, skin conditions, or ADHD, LGS might be to blame.

As a holistic doctor, I look for the underlying cause of a condition rather than just treat the symptoms. A conventional physician, on the other hand, simply prescribes a drug to treat the pathology he or she has diagnosed. Unfortunately, most drugs—I would estimate more than 90 percent—do not treat the underlying cause of an illness.

And what is the underlying cause of most illnesses? Most illnesses start in the gut. And if your gut isn't functioning right, it sets the stage for illness and disease. LGS is one of the most misdiagnosed conditions because doctors don't understand how much the food that we eat impacts our health. Even people with ulcers or colitis will be told that their condition will not improve by changing their diets, and they are given drugs instead. The truth is, everything we eat impacts our nutritional and hormonal balance. In the following chapters, I will explain how the gut—like the brain, heart, and liver—needs to be properly nourished in order for it to function correctly. Simply stated, if your gut is not healthy, your immune system is going to suffer. You will also learn the following:

- common symptoms of LGS
- what tests to ask your doctor for in order to correctly diagnose your condition

- the difference between good bacteria and bad bacteria
- what bacteria overgrowth in the gut reveals and how to use prebiotics and probiotics
- the best treatments and therapies for LGS-related conditions
- how to naturally correct hormone, mineral, and vitamin deficiencies
- lifestyle tips for optimal health
- the ideal diet for your gut and your overall health

Most people with chronic illnesses are suffering from gut issues, which is part of the reason they're sick, and traditional physicians don't understand what LGS is—much less how to diagnose and treat it. I estimate that more than 80 percent of people with chronic illnesses have leaky gut, an overgrowth of bad bacteria, or not enough good bacteria.

In addition to offering the best natural therapies and treatments to use for your particular health issues, I will provide stories about real-life patients I have successfully treated and tell you why many medications either don't work or make us sicker than we already are. For one thing, drug companies can't make natural substances like vitamins, but they can alter natural substances, making them foreign when they are absorbed into our systems. Because the body doesn't have a way to utilize or clear foreign substances in drugs, individuals will have adverse reactions. Knowing what I do now, it is not surprising that drug side effects are the number-three killer of people in the United States—it is estimated that more than 160,000 people die from adverse drug reactions annually.[1] In contrast, nutrients are very safe. There are zero deaths per year due to nutrient therapies that are naturally found in food and can be safely absorbed, utilized, and recycled in our bodies.

After twenty-five years of practicing holistic medicine, I can say without hesitation that improving your gut health and taking fewer drugs will help you feel better and look younger, improve your brain function, and treat myriad medical conditions. This book will give you all the information you need to change what you are now doing so you can have optimal gut health and, as a result, overall health and well-being. One caveat is that you must stick to the program! As you will soon discover, every time a patient consumes that forbidden sugary or salty treat they once craved, they literally can't stomach it. If you follow my advice, I promise you will feel like a new person (and you will lose some of those unwanted pounds—another positive side effect of treating your LGS).

I invite you to visit my website and blog at http://www.drbrownstein.com to get the latest updates on natural therapies and to let me know what's ailing you. I'd love to hear how your life has improved after reading this book and making the recommended changes and how you are finally able to enjoy each day pain- and worry-free.

To all our health!

David Brownstein, MD

Go with Your Gut
(Your Healthy Gut Checklist)

The future of medicine depends on doctors' willingness to listen, to use food and fitness as tools in pursuit of health, and to think outside the proverbial prescription and procedure box.

—Robynne Chutkan, MD, author of *Gutbliss* and
founder of the Digestive Center for Women

Before I get into the various conditions associated with leaky gut syndrome (LGS), I want to provide some basic information about your gut and give you pep and "prep" talk to prepare you for your journey to better health. Because every patient is different, there is no one-size-fits-all treatment, so you will need to see a health care provider (preferably a holistic one) to get a proper diagnosis and treatment regimen. The cases in this book will give you an idea about what is recommended to heal your leaky gut and the successful results that I have seen over the years.

The good news is that holistic treatments for LGS-related conditions (and every health issue, for that matter) are safer, faster, and longer lasting than most drug therapies. Like my father, you can see and feel the changes almost immediately, and if you stick to the program, the results can last a lifetime. Yet some of what I suggest, like changing your diet, will require intestinal fortitude. That's right—it takes guts to clean up your gut! Changing food habits is one of the hardest things for my patients to do, no matter how sick they are when they walk through my office door.

Refined sugar and salt that comes in so many of the products and foods we eat can be harder to kick than cigarettes for many people. And this is no accident. Food manufacturers understand the chemical changes that occur in your brain when you eat those sugary cereals, processed foods, or packaged desserts. The ingredients they put into their products are designed to get you hooked and craving more. Don't beat yourself up if you find it difficult to clean up your diet. You can wean yourself off forbidden foods rather than going cold turkey if you are struggling, and I will tell you the best foods and beverages to consume and what to avoid in "Your Healthy Gut Diet" on page 193. You will not feel deprived—in fact, you will feel revived. But make no mistake about it, your health and, in some cases, your life might depend on cleaning up your diet and balancing your nutritional and hormonal system. Here's what you need to know before you start.

Testing

When you go to your doctor for a checkup, he or she will take your weight and blood pressure, perhaps have you perform a lung capacity test, and do a complete blood count (CBC) to see whether levels of different substances in your blood fall within a normal range for your age, race, and gender. Your blood test results might fall outside the normal range for many reasons. Abnormal results might be a sign of a disorder or disease. Other factors—such as diet, menstrual cycle, physical activity level, alcohol intake, and medications (both prescription and over the counter [OTC])—can also cause abnormal results.

I do blood work-ups, which include checking for hormonal and nutritional levels, for all my patients, which helps me learn more about their general health and their gut health and find potential problems early. Your doctor should discuss your test results with you, especially if there are abnormalities.

Result Ranges for Common Blood Tests

Typical routine blood tests measure your red and white blood cell numbers as well as hemoglobin. This test can discover anemia, infection, inflammation, and even cancer. You can also get what's called a basic metabolic panel to check your heart, kidney, and liver function by looking at your blood glucose, calcium, and electrolyte levels. You might also have a lipoprotein panel that measures levels of fats in your blood, like "good" high-density lipoprotein (HDL) cholesterol, "bad" low-density lipoprotein (LDL) cholesterol, and triglycerides. The lab will usually include a notation on your test results if you fall into the abnormal range, so look for these red flags and discuss what the results mean with your doctor. Don't let "You're fine!" be the beginning and end of your conversation—

if there is something you don't understand, ask! (See "Ten Things Your Doctor Might Not Tell You" on page 15)

Test	Normal Range Results*
Red blood cell (varies with altitude)	Male: 5–6 million cells/mcL
	Female: 4–5 million cells/mcL
White blood cell	4,500–10,000 cells/mcL
Platelets	140,000–450,000 cells/mcL
Hemoglobin (varies with altitude)	Male: 14–17 gm/dl
	Female: 12–15 gm/dl
Hematocrit (varies with altitude)	Male: 41–50 percent
	Female: 36–44 percent
Mean corpuscular volume	80–95 femtoliter**

* cells/mcL = cells per microliter; gm/dl = grams per deciliter. Note: All values in this section are for adults only. Talk to your child's doctor about values on blood tests for children.

**A femtoliter is a measure of volume.

Blood Glucose

The following table shows the ranges for blood glucose levels after eight to twelve hours of fasting (not eating). It shows the normal range and the abnormal ranges, which are a sign of prediabetes or diabetes.

Plasma Glucose Results (mg/dl)*	Diagnosis
70–99	Normal
100–125	Prediabetes
126 and above	Diabetes**

* mg/dl = milligrams per deciliter.

** The test is repeated on another day to confirm the results.

Lipoprotein Panel

The table below shows ranges for total cholesterol, LDL cholesterol, and HDL cholesterol levels after nine to twelve hours of fasting. I will tell you more about cholesterol levels later on.

Total Cholesterol Level	Total Cholesterol Category
Less than 200 mg/dl	Desirable
200–239 mg/dl	Borderline high
240 mg/dl and above	High
LDL Cholesterol Level	**LDL Cholesterol Category**
Less than 100 mg/dl	Optimal
100–129 mg/dl	Near optimal/above optimal
130–159 mg/dl	Borderline high
160–189 mg/dl	High
190 mg/dl and above	Very high
HDL Cholesterol Level	**HDL Cholesterol Category**
Less than 40 mg/dl	A major risk factor for heart disease
40–59 mg/dl	The higher, the better
60 mg/dl and above	Considered protective against heart disease

Source: NIH.

Ten Things Your Doctor Might Not Tell You about Your Test Results

1. **Doctors sometimes skip the good news**. If your CBC, blood chemistry, and cholesterol results fall within normal ranges, the doctor's office probably won't call you about your lab report, or you will get a copy in the mail with little or no

explanation. Look over your results carefully and make a list of questions for when you talk to your doctor to follow up. Ask if there have been changes since the last test of the same type and what those changes mean.

2. **What's "normal" is different for men and women**. If you compare your blood test results with another person, you might be surprised to find differences depending on gender. For example, the normal range for the number of red blood cells in a CBC test is between five and six million cells per microliter for a man. The normal range is lower for women before menopause, between four and five million, likely because of blood loss during menstruation.

3. **Results can mean different things depending on your age**. Normal levels of hemoglobin vary by age—lower for children and higher for adults. Age matters for your cholesterol numbers too. Conventional wisdom is that most people, especially men over age forty-five and women over age fifty-five, should aim for LDL cholesterol levels of 160 to 190 mg/dl or above. But cholesterol is not the cause of heart disease, and cholesterol-lowering drugs (statins) have never been shown to significantly lower one's risk of developing heart disease. I will discuss the history of the high cholesterol/heart disease connection later on.

4. **A "positive" test result does not mean the news is good**. Some blood tests look for diseases by searching for molecular markers (DNA or protein) in your blood sample. Results are considered "positive" when the test finds the disease marker that it's looking for. In these cases, a positive test result means you might have the disease or disorder caused by LGS or something else.

5. **A "negative" test result is usually good news**. *Negative* does not mean "bad" when it comes to blood tests. A negative result tells you that the test did not detect what it was searching for, such as a disease marker or risk factor for a health condition.

When you've had a blood test to check for an infectious disease (hepatitis C, for example) getting back a negative result is a good thing because it means the test found no evidence of an infection.

6. **False-positive test results can happen**. That said, the first screening test for a condition often has to be checked by a second, more specific test to find out whether the results are accurate and will impact your health. So if you get a "positive" result on your first report, don't panic. Ask to be screened again and, if necessary, yet again to be certain that the results are correct. Although mix-ups of patient blood test samples are rare, they do happen.

7. **False-negative test results happen too**. Unfortunately, the reverse is also true; sometimes a test doesn't pick up evidence of a disease or condition even though you actually do have it. Using hepatitis C again as an example, the results can come back negative, but you might have been exposed to the virus several months ago and could be infected without knowing it. Getting another test is a good idea, especially if you are concerned that you were exposed to an infectious disease.

8. **Test values can differ from lab to lab**. A lab's reference range is based on test results from many people previously tested in that lab. What is considered a normal range might be different from another lab's results. If your prior blood test results vary from your latest report, it could be that your doctor sent the bloodwork to a different lab, so ask if you are unsure.

9. **Abnormal results might not be due to a disease**. A test result outside the normal range of expected lab results could lead to diagnosis of a disease or disorder. But there are other reasons that test outcomes can also be abnormal. If you ate a pastry before having a blood glucose test, drank alcohol the night before, or are taking certain medications, your result could be temporarily abnormal.

10. **Mistakes happen**. Although mix-ups of patient blood test samples are rare, they do happen, like the case reported on *ABC News* where an HIV patient's sample was accidentally switched with another patient's sample. The way your blood sample is handled by lab technicians before it's analyzed can also impact the results. Let's say the technician shakes the collection tube. This can cause the blood cells to break open, releasing their contents, which can potentially change the test results.

Dietary History

One of most important things I do when seeing a patient, aside from blood and other tests, is take a dietary history. When is the last time your primary-care doctor asked you about your diet? There are many diseases and illnesses that can't be diagnosed with bloodwork alone, so this is an essential part of determining whether a leaky gut is the cause of your complaint. I will ask my patients about everything they eat and drink—at breakfast, lunch, dinner, and snack time. The amount of water you consume is a vitally important part of your health (chances are, you are not drinking enough water, and there is an easy way to calculate how much you should be drinking for your body weight on page 25).

Most of my patients eat what's called the "standard American diet," also known as SAD because of how sick and unhealthy it makes people feel with its reliance on too many

Caveat: Health care professionals, including doctors, can make mistakes, so always be your own best advocate when it comes to your health! And don't be shy about questioning a lab result that doesn't seem right to you.

carbohydrates and the overconsumption of refined products (made primarily with refined sugar, grains, and flour). This diet causes nutrient deficiencies that can lead to a poorly functioning immune system and set the stage for LGS, which triggers the myriad conditions described in this book. Chapter 7 will explain how a balanced diet, with adequate amounts of protein, fats, and carbohydrates, can provide the body with the basic raw materials necessary to promote a healthy gut and immune system. It is the first line of defense against LGS and allows the healing process to begin.

The following is a sample of the dietary questionnaire that I give to my patients:

Dietary Questionnaire
- What do you eat for breakfast?
- What do you generally eat for lunch?
- What do you generally eat for dinner?
- What do you like to snack on?
- How much water do you drink per day, in ounces or glasses?
- Do you drink milk?
- How much coffee do you drink per day, in ounces?
- How much tea and what kind of tea do you drink per day?
- How many sodas per day do you drink?
- Do you drink fruit juice, and how much do you drink per day?
- How many alcoholic drinks per day do you drink?
- Do you have any food allergies and what are they?

Hair Tests: Detecting Nutritional Deficiencies

Another excellent way to determine whether my patients have a nutritional deficiency is through hair testing. The body is composed of many different minerals, and you can help ward off diseases and nutritional deficiency by making sure that your body has a healthy level of minerals and is free from toxins. Ask your doctor about a hair test to determine whether you have to make adjustments in your lifestyle and diet to cut out toxins or take supplements to correct a mineral deficiency. Here's how hair tests work and why they can help treat LGS:

- Your hair contains your medical history, much like your blood test results. The average head of hair has between 90,000 and 150,000 strands that grow ½ inch every month. Minerals and even toxins get deposited into the hair protein. The hair acts as a storage receptacle and gives me a biochemical record of a patient's nutritional status over a period of months. All that's needed is a strand of hair to determine whether a person has a nutritional deficiency. Hair testing allows me to see the bigger picture of my patients' overall health and underlying deficiencies. It's a noninvasive and economical way to determine the levels of minerals and to detect body toxins, and in some cases, it can be more accurate than blood or urine analyses.

Stool Test

I realize this sounds unpleasant, but a stool sample analysis, which is a series of tests of feces, is another excellent way to diagnose certain conditions affecting the digestive tract. These conditions include poor nutrient absorption due to LGS; infection from parasites, viruses, or bacteria; and cancer.

If you've never done one of these tests before, which should be part of any annual checkup, a stool sample can be taken at home in a clean container or using a collection swab kit that is mailed to a laboratory. The lab will do a microscopic examination and chemical and microbiologic tests that look for hidden (occult) blood, fat, fibers, bile, white blood cells, and sugars. The pH of the stool (potential of hydrogen that tells how acidic or alkaline a substance is) can also be measured. What's called a stool "culture" is also done to find out if bacteria are causing an infection.

Why Take This Test?
Stool analysis is done

- to identify diseases of the digestive tract, liver, and pancreas (Certain enzymes can be evaluated in the stool to help determine how well the pancreas is functioning.)
- to find the cause of symptoms affecting the digestive tract, including diarrhea, excess gas, nausea, vomiting, loss of appetite, bloating, abdominal pain, and cramping
- to check for poor absorption of nutrients by the digestive tract, a condition called malabsorption syndrome (For this test, stool samples are collected over a seventy-two-hour period and then checked for fat and sometimes for meat fibers [see sample below].)
- to determine the levels of good and bad bacteria as well as yeast and parasites

The following is a sample lab report form Genova Diagnostics, which I frequently use when testing my patients for leaky gut:

Patient: **SAMPLE PATIENT**
Age:
Sex:
MRN:

SAMPLE REPORT

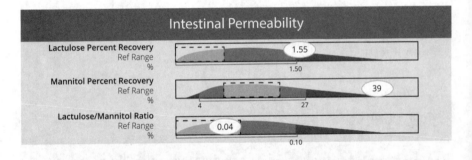

Intestinal Permeability

Lactulose Percent Recovery
Ref Range
%
1.55
1.50

Mannitol Percent Recovery
Ref Range
%
39
4   27

Lactulose/Mannitol Ratio
Ref Range
%
0.04
0.10

Commentary

The patient result for the "Before-Drink" sample was below the detection limit of assay (<0.08 mmol/L). Therefore, for the purpose of calculating the percent recovery of mannitol postchallenge, a value of 0.079 was used as the "Before-Drink" value of mannitol for the calculation.

This test has been developed and its performance characteristics determined by GSDL Inc. It has not been cleared or approved by the US Food and Drug Administration.

The **Reference Range** is a statistical interval representing 95 percent, or 2 standard deviations (SD) of the reference population.

One SD is a statistical interval representing 68 percent of the reference population. Values between 1 and 2 SD are not necessarily abnormal. Clinical correlation is suggested (see example below).

Result within Ref Range, but outside 1–80

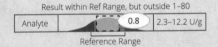

Analyte   0.8   2.3–12.2 U/g
Reference Range

Commentary is provided to the practitioner for educational purposes and should not be interpreted as diagnostic or treatment recommendations. Diagnosis and treatment decisions are the responsibility of the practitioner.

A stool digestive analysis helps identify whether patients are properly digesting their food. This test can check for the health of the intestines by identifying bacteria, both good and bad, as well as the presence of parasites and yeast. Once all this information is gathered, a treatment plan can be instituted to help the gut become healthier. This leads to better digestion and an improved immune system because more than half of the immune system cells reside in the intestines.

How to Prepare

To best prepare for this test, you should avoid certain medicines. You might need to stop taking medicines such as antacids, antidiarrheals, antiparasitics, antibiotics, laxatives, or NSAIDs for one to two weeks prior to the test. Make sure you tell your doctor about all the nonprescription and prescription medicines you take before doing any tests. As with any test, talk to your doctor about what you need to do to prepare and what the results mean.[1]

Upper Gastrointestinal Series

These tests are usually performed by a gastroenterologist, who specializes in UGI problems (see Chapter 2 on digestive distress). The tests allow the doctor to examine the upper and middle sections of the gastrointestinal tract using barium contrast material (a liquid form of soft, silvery metallic alkaline) and fluoroscopy (medical imaging that shows an X-ray video on a monitor).

Before the test, you drink a mixture of barium and water. The barium is sometimes combined with gas-making crystals. Your doctor then watches the movement of the barium through your esophagus, stomach, and the small intestine on a screen. Several X-ray pictures are taken at different times and from different views.

Note: You do not have to have this test unless you are exhibiting these symptoms.

A follow-up can be done immediately after a UGI to look at the rest of the small intestine. If just the throat and esophagus are being looked at, you will have what's called an esophagram (or barium swallow). Another way to look at the lining of the esophagus, stomach, and upper small intestine is by doing an upper endoscopy using a thin, flexible tube (endoscope).

Why Have a UGI Series?

A UGI series is done

- to diagnose LGS, inflamed areas of the intestine, or problems with the squeezing motion that moves food through the intestines (See section on acid reflux on page 41.)
- if you have trouble swallowing or are vomiting, burping up food, or experiencing belly pain or indigestion.
- to find narrow spots in the upper intestinal tract, ulcers, tumors, polyps, or pyloric stenosis (the narrowing of the opening from the stomach to the first part of the small intestine)
- to find swallowed objects[2]

Basic LGS Treatment

I cover a number of conditions and illnesses in this book, for which the treatments vary depending on a patient's case history and test results. That said, there are general lifestyle and dietary changes that everyone with LGS symptoms can make to kick-start the healing process. You can refer to the chapters describing your particular health issue for full details on what kinds of treatments I typically use to heal a leaky gut. If you read no farther than this page, here's what I want you to do starting today.

Drink More Water

Whatever amount of water you drink a day, if you are drinking it at all, it is probably not enough. The one common denominator in just about every patient I see is dehydration, a leading cause of digestive and other problems. The amount of coffee, soda, and juice you drink does not count. The beverage of choice is water, which is free at most restaurants (if not bottled) and still thankfully abundant. There has been some confusion in the media and among health officials about the number of glasses one should drink a day, and Table 1 contains an easy calculation that will tell you exactly how much is needed for your weight:

Table 1: Weight/Water Calculation

Take your weight in pounds.

Divide the weight in half.

The result is the number of ounces of water you should drink daily.

For a 130-pound woman, that's 65 ounces, or about 8 cups. It makes sense that we need to drink more water because the human body is 60 percent water, while the brain is about 70 percent water. (Body composition varies according to gender and fitness level, because fatty tissue contains less water than lean tissue.) In addition to drinking enough water for your individual body, everyone should

- cut out soda, including diet soda, reduce coffee intake (it's dehydrating), and eliminate juice, which is mostly sugar
- avoid refined sugar, salt, white flour products, vegetable and soy oils, and processed "junk" food
- eat a plant-based, whole-food "Paleo" diet with lots of colorful fruits and veggies (more on this later)
- avoid animal products where the animals were fed hormones and raised in inhumane environments
- lose excess weight to achieve the right body mass index (BMI) for your height, age, and gender. (This will happen if you follow the advice above.)
- enjoy mindful eating techniques rather than a fast-food, "mindless" eating mentality

Full details are in Chapter 7, "The Healthy Gut Diet." This is usually the point where my patients tell me, "But I can't give up my [fill in the blank]!" To this, I say, "Can you give up your bloated belly, heartburn, muscle and joint pain, fatigue, foggy brain, heartburn, rashes, allergies, or depression?" If you'd rather be uncomfortable or in pain than symptom-free—living your life to the fullest and still being around to watch your children graduate, walk down the aisle, and have their own children—you will make the appropriate dietary changes.

Here are some basic facts and diagrams that might help you on your journey to health and well-being:

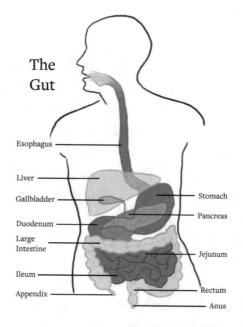

The Gut

Esophagus

Liver

Gallbladder

Duodenum

Large Intestine

Ileum

Appendix

Stomach

Pancreas

Jejunum

Rectum

Anus

Colon and Rectum
(Large Bowel)

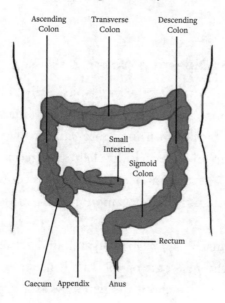

Ascending Colon

Transverse Colon

Descending Colon

Small Intestine

Sigmoid Colon

Rectum

Caecum   Appendix   Anus

What Is the Gut?

The gut, or the intestine, is the place where most of the nutrients and water are absorbed into the body. When we eat, food passes down the esophagus, into the stomach, and then into the small intestine. The gut processes food from the time it is first eaten until it is either absorbed by the body or passed out as stools (feces). Digestion actually begins in the mouth, where your teeth and chemicals made by the body's enzymes break down food. Muscular contractions help move food in the esophagus down into the stomach.

Chemicals produced by cells in the stomach do most of the work of digestion. While some foods and liquids are absorbed through the lining of the stomach, much is absorbed in the small intestine. Muscles in the wall of the gut mix your food with the enzymes produced by the body. They also move food along toward the end of the gut. Food that can't be digested turns into waste, bacteria, and undigested food, which are passed out as feces.

How Does Digestion Work?

The mouth contains salivary glands. Saliva lubricates food and contains chemicals (enzymes) that digest your meal. Your teeth break down food into smaller pieces. Saliva also contains special chemicals that help stop germs from causing infections. The amount of saliva released is controlled by your nervous system. A certain amount of saliva is continuously released.

The stomach is a *J*-shaped organ found between the esophagus and the first part of the small intestine (duodenum). When empty, it is about the same size as a large sausage. Its main function is to help digest the food you eat. The other main function of the stomach is to store food until the gut is ready to receive it.

Digestion involves breaking food down into its most basic parts. It is absorbed through the wall of the gut into the bloodstream and transported around the body. Simply chewing food doesn't release essential nutrients—enzymes are needed for this. The wall of the stomach has several different layers. The inner layers contain special glands. These glands release enzymes, hormones, acid, and other substances. These secretions form gastric juice, the liquid found in the stomach, muscle, and other tissue from the outer layers. A few minutes after food enters the stomach, the muscles within the stomach wall start to contract. This creates gentle waves in the stomach contents that mix the food with gastric juice. Using its muscles, the stomach then pushes small amounts of food (now known as chyme) into the duodenum. The stomach has two sphincters, one at the bottom and one at the top. Sphincters are bands of muscles that form a ring. This stops chyme from going into the duodenum before it is ready.

Digestion of food is controlled by your brain, nervous system, and various hormones released in the gut. Even before you begin eating, signals from your brain travel from nerves to your stomach. This causes gastric juice to be released in preparation for food arriving. Once food reaches the stomach, special cells that detect changes in the body's receptors send signals that release more gastric juice and cause more muscular contractions.

The small intestine, which is twenty feet long, has three parts: the duodenum, jejunum, and ileum. Cells and glands in the lining of the small intestines also produce intestinal juice

Details around
Pancreas

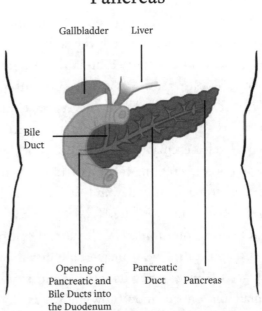

Gallbladder   Liver

Bile
Duct

Opening of   Pancreatic
Pancreatic and   Duct   Pancreas
Bile Ducts into
the Duodenum

that aids digestion. Contractions in the wall of the small intestine help mix food and move it along.

The small intestine also has special features that increase the amount of nutrients absorbed by the body. The inner layer of the small intestine has millions of villi, tiny fingerlike structures with small blood vessels inside. These are covered by a thin layer of cells, which allow nutrients released by digestion to enter the blood. Most of the important nutrients needed by the body are absorbed at different points of the small intestine.

The inside of the large intestine (five feet long) is wider than the small intestine. It does not contain villi and mainly absorbs water. Bacteria in the large intestine also help with the final stages of digestion. Once chyme has been in the large intestine for several hours, it becomes semisolid because most of the water has been removed. These remnants are known as stools and are excreted through the anus. This long and winding road from mouth to south takes about twelve hours.

A Miniglossary of Gut and Other Body Terms

Here are a few biological terms that you should become familiar with while reading the upcoming chapters.

Bacteria (Good)

Most bacteria are harmless to humans, and some are even beneficial. Good, or symbiotic, bacteria not only help with digestion but also help produce vitamins and protect you against bad bacteria. In many ways, bacteria help sustain life for humans. Certain bacteria are safe in food, and those found in fermented foods can help people with LGS. Good bacteria, such as *Lactobacillus rhamnosus*, have been shown to enhance the immune system. They also form a barrier to help protect us from bad bacteria by altering acidity level or by releasing toxins that harm the bad bacteria.[3]

Bacteria (Bad)

Pathogenic, or bad, bacteria can produce problems ranging from the mild to fatal, including food poisoning, a toothache, and death. Some bacteria such as Salmonella can cause a brief bout of stomachache or diarrhea, which, in some severe cases, can be deadly. Up to 30 percent of the protein and carbs you eat enter your colon, where your gut bacteria break them down, according to the journal of *Nutrition in Clinical Practice*. But just a few days of eating a high-fat diet can disrupt the balance of good and bad bacteria in your system, throwing off your digestive process.[4]

Enzymes

There are 2,709 different types of enzymes working in the human body. Amylase enzymes are used in digestion to break down food into simple chemicals, such as the starch in potatoes or bread. They are made from twisted proteins that help run our metabolism, and some mix with our saliva to help the teeth soften food. If our digestion is out of whack, like when we're on vacation or when we are stressed, a digestive enzyme supplement can hit the spot. These little gut helpers work just like your body's own enzymes to help break down food so you can absorb nutrients more easily.

Gut Flora

Gut microbiota (a.k.a. gut flora) is the name given to the microorganisms that live in the intestine. Our gut flora contains tens of trillions of microorganisms, including at least one thousand different species of recognized bacteria (most gut flora is still unknown) with more than three million genes (150 times more than human genes).[5]

Hormones

Hormones are produced by glands in several areas of the body, including the thyroid, the largest hormone gland. They are chemical messengers that work with the nervous system to help regulate the body's functions. The term comes from the Greek word *horman*, meaning "to set in motion." Hormones play a role in how we sleep, our moods, and how we mature into adulthood. There are one hundred hormones in the body, the most well known being insulin, adrenaline, testosterone, and estrogen.

Immune System

The immune system is the body's protection system, which keeps it free from disease. Its cells clean out any invaders, such as bacteria and viruses.

Mitochondria

Mitochondria are tiny torpedo-shaped power plants that work inside every cell to release energy for your body. They even carry their own supply of DNA. They burn food to make a superfuel called adenosine triphosphate (ATP; the chemical used to store energy in cells). When our cells need a boost, our bodies smash apart the ATPs, which unleash flashes of life-giving energy (five million ATPs are made every second). The leftover pieces are recycled into new ATPs.

Prebiotics

Prebiotics nourish good bacteria by letting them flourish in a healthy environment. They are present in fermented foods. Some examples include yogurt, kefir, sauerkraut, and kimchi. Store-bought yogurts, however, are not usually effective because they are loaded with sugar, but you can make your own.

Probiotics

Gut flora, or microbiota, is an intricate community of microorganisms in the digestive tract. Their presence in our intestines has several benefits, such as collecting energy from short-chain fatty acids. People have approximately one hundred million intestinal microorganisms, much more than the total number of cells in the human body. Microorganisms are like nutrient-rich sanctuaries. We can "repopulate" the gut with large amounts of live bacteria using probiotics, which are live strains of bacteria that can be taken in pill, powder, or liquid form. One probiotic strain, GanedenBC30, which is added to a wide range of food products, has been found to help your body break down proteins. Probiotic supplements provide good bacteria for the gut. It can also increase the number of good microorganisms. Your doctor can help you choose which particular type is best for you.

Villi

The primary function of the villi in the small intestine is to increase the absorption of nutrients from food passing through the small intestine.

Now that you know how the digestive process works, the next chapter will explain what happens to our health when there are disruptions in the gut and things go haywire.

Digestive Distress

All disease begins in the gut.

—Hippocrates

Hippocrates, the father of Western medicine, understood the importance of the gut health, and this understanding is just as valuable today as it was two thousand years ago. While not all illnesses begin in the gut (genetic conditions, for example), there is evidence that most chronic diseases do start there. The reason, as I explained earlier, has to do with the different gut bacteria in our digestive tracts and the condition of the gut lining. It is also important to know that the largest concentration of immune system cells resides in the gut.

Numerous studies have shown that unwanted bacterial products called endotoxins and food proteins can either be carried into the blood along with dietary fat or leak past the tight cell junctions that are supposed to prevent unwanted substances from crossing the gut lining. When this happens, our immune system mounts an attack against these foreign molecules (like an army responding to an invasion from a hostile country), resulting in chronic inflammation and immune dysregulation that can wreak havoc over time. The chronic inflammation can lead to autoimmune disorders, as the immune system can't defend antibodies from attacking its own tissues. In fact, leaky gut syndrome (LGS) is one of the leading causes of diet-induced chronic inflammation.

What Is Inflammation and Why Should You Care?

Before I go into the various digestive problems that are the result of a poor diet, nutritional imbalances, and LGS, let me briefly explain what inflammation is. It involves many cells and hundreds of different molecules, all of which communicate in complex ways. Cells communicate with one another by producing cytokines (proteins that signal cells) and other molecules that tell a neighboring cell what is going on. When the cytokines are inflammatory in nature, the cell is telling its neighbors that there is danger nearby. This can mean that the cell has encountered an infectious agent, or the cell might have come into contact with a food protein that should not be in the bloodstream. The body responds to these items by producing more inflammatory molecules that puts the immune system into overdrive to destroy the foreign substance. Simply put, inflammation is the response of the immune system to foreign invaders, toxins, or even cell injury. The purpose of inflammation is to stimulate the immune system to rectify problems.

Let's say you stub your toe on a chair, and your toe becomes red, warm, swollen, and painful. The discolored, warm skin and obviously deformed toe is a perfect example of short-term inflammation at work. It's the body's way of beginning to heal itself—in this case, by recruiting inflammatory cells to stimu-late the healing process. Other cells are brought in to repair the injured tissue and replace it with healthy tissue. When the healing process is completed, the toe goes back to its normal size and shape. Without the inflammatory response, pathogens like bacteria and viruses could easily run rampant.

But there is another type of inflammation that can be dan-gerous when deployed against the body's healthy cells. Auto-immune disorders are examples of the body inadvertently attacking its own tissues by producing antibodies. Autoimmune disorders are characterized by the production of antibodies and usually occur when there is a systemic (whole body) inflam-mation present. LGS can lead to autoimmune disorders by allowing foreign substances to cross the gut membrane, which stimulates the body to produce antibodies. Many times, these foreign substances have similar properties to our own cells, and the immune system can mistakably produce antibodies against its own cells.

At the end of day, systemic inflammation caused by LGS might be the missing link between digestive distress, obesity, and many of the chronic diseases, including autoimmune dis-orders, that are making us sick (see Chapter 3 on autoimmune diseases).

The Gut-Wrenching Facts

There are trillions of bacteria in the gut, collectively known as the gut flora. Some of these bacteria are our friends—others are not. The number and composition of gut bacteria can affect our physical and mental health. For example, during an acute bac-terial infection such as pneumonia, they can lead to fever and aches and pains, as well as mental changes such as depression and anxiety. You see, many bacteria produce endotoxins, which are created by toxic bacteria that can cause inflammation of the gut and many other tissues in the body.

More and more studies have correlated dietary habits to inflammation. It's quite simple, really—a diet can be inflammatory (unhealthy) or anti-inflammatory (healthy). In this chapter and throughout this book, I will provide information about which foods to eat, which foods and ingredients to avoid, and which supplements and other remedies you can take to help treat your particular condition and ease your discomfort. Your immune system and your gut are very responsive to your diet. Eating healthy foods nourishes the body's tissues, while eating unhealthy food produces inflammation and can lead to chronic disease. Your best bet is to live a healthy lifestyle, eat the right foods, steer clear of the inflammatory-provoking ones in the typical Western diet, and get adequate amounts of water, exercise, and restorative sleep.

A whole-food-based diet that supplies the body with the nutrients it needs is the best option for gut and overall health. A healthy diet that includes prebiotic ingredients (substances that nourish the body's natural gut bacteria) as well as other vitamins and minerals *should* be the standard American diet. Unfortunately, this is not the case in our modern world, where most people eat a standard American diet filled with nutrient-depleting refined foods that leave the body deficient and imbalanced in essential nutrients and good bacteria. A probiotic supplement, which contains beneficial gut bacteria, can help the gastrointestinal tract maintain optimal levels of healthy bacteria. Adequate amounts of healthy bacteria will reduce inflammation in the gut and in the rest of the body. Probiotic foods such as unsweetened yogurt with active, live cultures of beneficial bacteria, as well as kefir and sauerkraut—healthy fermented foods—can also help (see "Your Healthy Gut Diet" on page 193).

Like an engine in need of high-grade fuel in order to run smoothly, our bodies need food that fuels them with the right raw materials—vitamins, minerals, protein, and fat—so they can function optimally. Our cells thrive on the nutrients extracted from the foods like these to produce the energy and essential oxygen and minerals that they need to live. That said, much can go wrong during that trip down the digestive highway, and the following conditions are some of the most common problems that can occur along the way.

Breaking Your Heartburn

Most of us have experienced heartburn (a.k.a. acid reflux) at one time or another—perhaps after eating greasy food. It occurs when acid from the stomach rises up into the esophagus, the muscular structure that carries food from the mouth to the stomach. It's important to understand how the stomach works. The gastric cells that line the stomach produce hydrochloric acid, which is used to digest food. The stomach has a mucous lining to protect it from this acid, but the esophagus does not. The sphincter at the bottom of the esophagus helps separate the stomach contents from the esophagus contents. When people are overweight, their abdominal fat can continually push stomach contents up into the esophagus, which can cause acid to be released into the esophagus. Once acid enters the esophagus, it can result in burning and pain that can go from the front of the belly all the way up the breast bone of the chest.

Additionally, if stomach contents are continually pushed up into the esophagus, the acid can weaken the esophageal sphincter over time. The technical term for this is condition is a hiatal hernia. Stomach acid can cause the esophagus to burn and even bleed. Persistent acid irritation to the esophagus can turn normal esophageal cells into cancer cells. This is known as Barrett's esophagus.

Gastroesophageal reflux disease (GERD) is a condition in which stomach acid enters the esophagus and damages the esophageal lining. Conventional medicine's approach to GERD is to block stomach acid production. That would be fine if the cause of GERD was too much stomach acid production, but this is not true in most cases. Stomach acid is being appropriately produced to digest food; in the case of GERD, it is inappropriately delivered to the esophagus.

When treating GERD, conventional medicine uses what's called proton-pump inhibitors (PPIs), such as Prilosec and Nexium, which are potent acid-blocking drugs. While these medications might provide temporary relief,

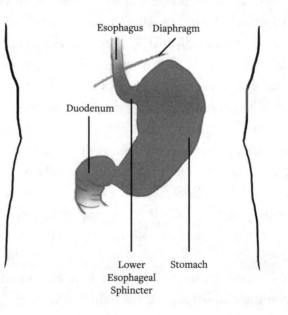

they work by poisoning an enzyme in the stomach's gastric cells so it stops producing hydrochloric acid. In effect, PPIs are perfect drugs to block the stomach's natural production of hydrochloric acid. But because you can't properly digest food without stomach acid, PPIs set off a chain reaction down the rest of the intestinal tract. This can result in bacterial overgrowth and poor absorption of nutrients in the intestines. When the intestines become imbalanced from dysbiotic (imbalance) bacteria, a host of problems develop, including

- an inability to absorb nutrients,
- imbalanced gut flora, and
- leaky gut membranes.

Treatments for Acid Reflux and GERD

The burning in the esophagus and stomach is like a fire. How do you put out fire? You use water, of course. You need to drink an adequate amount of water between meals (see Table 1 in Chapter 1). Sadly, most people with GERD do not drink enough water to douse the fire in their bellies, and it is impossible to overcome GERD if they do not drink adequate amounts of water. It's also important to avoid drinking too much water during mealtime, as this will dilute normal stomach acid and interfere with proper digestion.

Acid-blocking drugs can provide symptom relief from GERD, but they do not treat the underlying causes. And their long-term use is fraught with serious adverse effects. I only use acid-blocking drugs when absolutely necessary. And if I use them at all, it's for the shortest time period possible—no more than a few weeks. In addition to putting out the acid reflux fire with water, you need to do the following:

- **Clean up your diet**. Eat a high-protein or "Paleo" diet and avoid sugar, salt, and grains.
- **Lose weight**. Following the Leaky Gut Diet combined with physical activity is the best and fastest way to lose weight.
- **Drink aloe vera juice**. Taking aloe vera (2–4 tablespoons four times a day) can sooth the esophagus and help it heal from reflux.

Causes of GERD

There is usually no single cause of GERD, but the most common factors are alcohol use, poor diet, obesity, pregnancy, dehydration, and smoking.

Symptoms of GERD

Signs and symptoms include

- a burning sensation in your chest (heartburn), sometimes spreading to your throat, along with a sour taste in your mouth
- chest pain
- difficulty swallowing
- dry cough
- hoarseness or sore throat
- regurgitation of food or sour liquid (acid reflux)
- sensation of a lump in your throat

Keep in mind that spicy and fried foods, citrus, chocolate, and caffeine can all make these symptoms worse.[1]

Peter's Story

Peter, a fifty-eight-year-old auto executive, was diagnosed with GERD six months before coming to see me. His doctor did an esophageal gastroduodenoscopy (a scope test) and put him on Prilosec, which he was told to stay on for the rest of his life. When he saw me, he was still suffering from GERD symptoms, although he was feeling a bit better with the Prilosec. He had read my book *Drugs That Don't Work and Natural Therapies That Do!* and didn't want to take the acid-blocking drug forever, as he was worried about the long-term side effects.

As I do with all new patients, I performed a dietary history and physical exam. Peter was eating a standard American diet filled with refined food, fatty foods, several sodas, and several cups a coffee a day, all of which gave him a leaky gut. Peter's dietary choices were not providing him with the nutrients his body needed to optimally function; in fact, he was deficient in many essential nutrients. Peter was about forty pounds overweight and eating from the time he got home from work until bedtime. His stomach was large and tender, and the top was pushing up into his esophagus, which I could feel by palpating (poking around with my fingers). He also smoked two packs of cigarettes a day. I reset his stomach's position by manually pulling it down. He felt immediately better, but I explained that his pain and GERD would return if he didn't lose weight and change his lifestyle, as the abdominal fat would eventually push the stomach back up into the esophageal opening.

I told him to start with a goal of losing fifteen pounds, which would make a huge difference, even though he needed to lose forty pounds. He had to cut out fatty foods and refined flour and salt, drink half his body weight (in ounces) in water, and eat whole foods. He needed to stop smoking because it decreases the tone of the esophageal sphincter (aside from the other health hazards). Had had to exercise by simply moving—I don't always tell my patients to go to the gym because I know many won't do it. Peter was also using Tums, an antacid, in between taking Prilosec, which worked temporarily, but he was still waking up at night in agony. He was further motivated to make these lifestyle changes because an earlier test showed that his esophageal cells were becoming precancerous, and he was diagnosed with Barrett's esophagus.

Peter listened to my advice and cut back on the coffee, ate better, and started walking up to thirty minutes a day. When I saw him for a follow-up visit six weeks later, he was feeling and looking better. He wasn't using Tums and had lost five pounds, but he was still taking Prilosec. His stool tests showed LGS, which was causing nutrient imbalances. I found Peter very low in vitamin B12 (hydroxocobalamin), which is common in people taking acid-blocking medications. I taught Peter to inject 1 mg of natural vitamin B12 twice weekly. The B12 helped clear up his constipation, diarrhea, and bloating after meals.

A month later, he came back again after losing fifteen pounds. At this point, I tapered him off the Prilosec. Three months later, he was like a new man. His GERD and LGS were gone. He told me he felt like a million bucks and that his family and friends all told him he looked fantastic. He vowed to take care of himself from then on—which he did.

Go Away from the Burn

If you are suffering from heartburn or other symptoms of acid reflux, I suggest making the following simple changes to your diet and lifestyle:

Weaning Off Prilosec

Never stop taking medications cold turkey. In the case of acid-blocking drugs, you must "titrate" off, which means gradually weaning yourself off the medication. If you suddenly stop these medications, you can get a rebound excess stomach acid production, which can exacerbate GERD symptoms. This is true for many prescription drugs.

To stop taking Prilosec (or any acid-blocking drug), start by taking another antacid drug like Zantac and Tagamet (150 mg daily) while continuing with the Prilosec. After so many weeks, cut down to a half a pill every three days. It can take up to twelve weeks to get off an acid-blocking drug completely.

1. **Eat a real "happy" meal instead of a SAD one.** Eliminate refined and processed foods from your diet and replace them with lean, high-protein foods. For example, try a certified humane, free-range chicken breast without skin and antibiotics. Or try grass-fed (not factory) meat instead of deep-fried chicken, pasta, or rice.
2. **Downsize.** Eat more frequently but cut down on your portions. Smaller meals and healthy bridge snacks (such as organic nuts) are easier on your stomach.
3. **Stop eating before you're too full.** Americans like large portions, but it's better for your health (and for

weight control) if you eat slower and stop before you feel stuffed. Too much food can expand the stomach and cause its acidic contents to rise into the esophagus. We sometimes don't feel sated until fifteen or twenty minutes after we finish our meal. Eating too much food can worsen GERD symptoms if the stomach is pushed up into the esophagus.

4. **Avoid your triggers**. Pay attention to the foods and drinks that bring on your heartburn or make it worse. These can include
   - coffee or tea (both regular and decaffeinated)
   - soda and other carbonated or caffeinated beverages
   - alcohol
   - citrus fruits, such as oranges and lemons
   - tomatoes and products that are made with tomatoes, such as tomato sauce and salsa
   - chocolate
   - mint or peppermint
   - fatty or spicy foods, such as chili or curry
   - onions and garlic

5. **Sleep it off**. Did you know you can reduce your acid reflux while you sleep? Here's how:

   Raise the head of your bed 4–6 inches. The elevation will help keep your stomach contents down. You can do this by putting blocks under the legs of your bed (just using big pillows won't work because it will put more pressure on your belly). Don't eat for at least two or three hours before going to sleep.

6. **Loosen up**. Don't wear tight, form-fitting clothes and take your belt out a notch or two. Extra pressure around your belly can push your stomach up and make your acid reflux spike.

7. **Lose it**. If you're overweight or obese like Peter was, dropping those extra pounds can also take the pressure off.

8. **Stop smoking**. Do I really have to tell you this? If you smoke, stop. Aside from myriad health risks, smoking creates more stomach acid, and cigarettes negatively affect the lower esophageal sphincter, which makes it more difficult to keep that acid down where it belongs. Ask your doctor for help if you have tried and failed to quit on your own.

9. **Move it!** You don't have to be a gym rat or marathon runner to reap the benefits of physical activity. As I always tell my patients, walking counts as exercise, and moving in any way that you can is great for you from head to toe. Engaging in physical activity that you enjoy will keep you feeling young and healthy (and help get your bowels moving properly).[2]

Irritable Bowel Syndrome

Irritable bowel syndrome (IBS) is a common problem that affects the large intestine. The symptoms are the same as LGS—abdominal cramping, bloating, and irregularity. Some people with IBS have constipation, while others can have diarrhea. And yet others can alternate between the two. IBS can cause a great deal of discomfort, although it does not pose a danger to the intestines or stomach. IBS affects about twice as many women as men, and it is frequently found in people younger than age forty-five.[3]

Treatments for IBS
My experience has clearly shown that the cause of IBS can be multifactorial. However, the most common reasons people

develop IBS are LGS, food allergies, and/or bacterial, fungal, yeast, or parasite overgrowths. When substances get absorbed into your gut that shouldn't be there due to LGS, antibodies and other inflammatory molecules are produced. This is why the first thing I do with my IBS patients is take a complete dietary history. Inevitably, I find that they are eating an unhealthy diet that consists of too many refined foods that lack in basic minerals, nutrients, and good bacteria (flora) that our stomachs need to function optimally. Dairy and gluten are the worst foods for most people with IBS.

Dairy and gluten are two of the most common trigger foods. In far too many patients, they can cause inflammation of the gut cells, which often leads to the leaking of food proteins across the gut barrier. This causes the body to produce antibodies against these food proteins, leading to a food allergy. The bloating and discomfort you feel after eating will go away simply by eating the right diet and correcting imbalances in the gut with prebiotics and probiotics (see page 33).

Another factor that can lead to IBS is an infection of the gut. This can also take the form of an abnormal overgrowth of bacteria, yeast, viruses, and parasites. You must also lower the amounts of bad bacteria, yeast, and parasites, if present, which can be done with herbal and vitamin supplements. If you get IBS, increase your intake of vitamin C temporarily to allow the leaky gut to seal up again.

You can start by avoiding gluten, dairy, and processed foods for six weeks to see if you get better. The reason being, antibodies can continue to circulate in your system for up to six weeks after you consume something, so you have to wait until they are all gone to see if your symptoms are better. If you fall off the food wagon before the end of six weeks, you have to start over. At the same time, supply the gut with the right nutrients to correct any imbalances (ask your holistic doctor to test for deficiencies). I also check for food allergies with blood tests and encourage stress management because anxiety makes IBS worse.

Fizzle Out Your GERD and IBS

Seltzer might seem like a good alternative to sugary sodas and juice, but it can cause heartburn in some people. Carbonated water can increase gas and bloating in the stomach and trigger acid reflux. People with GERD or IBS might notice that seltzer brings on these symptoms. Additionally, flavored fizzy water contains citric acid, which can be especially damaging. Try adding a lime, cucumber, or mint to plain water instead. Club soda has added sodium and sweeteners, so phase out the fizz if you want to start feeling better.

Richard's Story

Richard was an eighty-eight-year-old retired salesman who looked about sixty. He played tennis twice a week and tried to take care of himself. His biggest complaint was his stomach. He felt bloated and experienced stomach pain after every meal, and he had both constipation and diarrhea that lasted for four weeks several times a year. He had seen several gastroenterologists who gave him endoscope tests and was told by his doctors that everything looked fine before they put him on antacid drugs. He didn't want to take the drugs, so he saw me for a second opinion.

After a dietary history, I found that he was eating a large amount of dairy in the form of yogurt because he thought it was good for his gut. When I told him that most store-bought yogurts are loaded with sugar and are not healthy, he went home and read the labels. He saw, in fact, that the yogurts he was eating contained up to 40 grams of sugar, which is similar to the amount in a can of soda. Many people like Richard have dairy sensitivities, which are also common in the elderly. I did a blood food allergy test as well as a stool analysis and diagnosed him with LGS. I told Richard that his symptoms would not go away unless he changed his diet. He was found to have high antibody levels to casein, the main protein in cow's milk products.

I told him to immediately cut out dairy. At the same time, I corrected the nutritional imbalances found in his tests with the proper supplements. When he came back six months later, he was completely recovered and has been nearly IBS- and LGS-free ever since. When he did get the occasional episode, however—usually triggered from eating something he should not be eating—he found that eating a semisweet pickle would settle his stomach down. Pickles, which are fermented, have anti-inflammatory effects (I'll discuss more about this later on). Richard was so pleased by this discovery that brought me a bottle of pickles the next time he came for a physical.

Constipation

Constipation is more of a symptom than a condition and can be caused by inflammation and imbalances in the gut. The symptoms are difficulty passing stools, straining, hard stools, and having fewer bowel movements (less than one time a day). This is one of the most common digestive complaints, with approximately sixty million people in the United States having constipation at some point in their lives. Constipation also can alternate with diarrhea when you have IBS.

Causes of Constipation

There are several causes of constipation, including IBS; LGS; stress; lack of exercise; a diet high in refined carbohydrates and low in fruits, vegetables, and fiber; and sudden lifestyle changes. Being over- or underweight can also be a factor. An underactive thyroid gland, which can go undetected by standard blood tests, is another common cause. Ignoring the urge to have a bowel movement can also bring on constipation. Waiting too long to defecate can bring on what's called fecal impaction—doctors can refer to patients with this as being "full of it." It's no laughing matter, however, because severe cases can result in a trip to the emergency room.

What Is the Normal Number of Times to Go to the Bathroom?

When it comes to the number of trips you make to the bathroom to evacuate, every individual is different. Some people go once a day, others more than once, while some defecate only a few times a week. That said, it is optimal to move your bowels at least once per day. One of my mentors, Dr. Majid Ali, said that two to four effortless, odorless bowel movements per day are optimal. If you're feeling bloated and uncomfortable for longer than a few days, it's best to see your doctor.

Treatments for Constipation

Drinking adequate amounts of water as well as getting refined foods and sugars out of your diet will usually solve the problem quickly. Additionally, eating whole foods, including fruits and vegetables, will provide you with the natural fiber you need to get things moving. Over-the-counter (OTC) laxatives such as Miralax, generic powders that contain Polyethylene glycol, or pills with bisacodyl USP (in Dulcolax and other products) will create a loss of nutrients and minerals if taken regularly. Do not take these for long periods of time, as these substances can be addictive, making it impossible for you to have a normal bowel movement without them.

In addition to getting rid of refined foods through dietary changes, ask your doctor to test for nutritional imbalances or food allergies that need to be corrected. Vitamin C is also an excellent treatment for constipation. It is an essential nutrient and we'd die without it. Humans can't produce their own, but you can get it from fruits and vegetables. If you don't get enough, and most people don't, I suggest 3,000 to 5,000 mg of vitamin C and 100 to 400 mg of magnesium at bedtime, which will take care of more than 95 percent of people suffering from constipation.

The best form of vitamin C to take when you are suffering from constipation is buffered vitamin C powder. In these cases, I suggest using about 5,000 mg twice daily along with taking 100 to 400 mg/day of magnesium at bedtime.

Be Water Wise at Mealtime

I know it seems counterintuitive, especially when drinking more water is a critical part of treating LGS-related conditions, but drinking too much water during meals can actually impede digestion. Water dilutes the digestive acids that help breakdown of food and eliminate infectious agents that might be ingested along with food. A rule of thumb for mealtime is to drink most of your daily water at least thirty minutes before you eat and wait at least one hour after you finish before drinking any more. Here are some other tips for being water wise:

1. **Take small sips.** If you like to have a little liquid when you eat, take small sips during your meal. Not only does this cleanse your palate, you will feel hydrated without flooding the digestive system at the time it is working its hardest. Try adding a squeeze of lemon or a bit of apple cider vinegar to your water to keep the digestive process running smoothly.

2. **Choose warm over cold.** Iced drinks during meals can be a problem for those with digestive issues. The body has to actively warm the liquid, which uses energy. If you want to sip something at mealtime, room-temperature or warm liquids such as green, black, or white tea are more gut-friendly. Warm broths are also an excellent option and can actually aid digestion.

Diarrhea

The other most common digestive distress is diarrhea, which I probably don't have to tell you is when stools are loose and watery. The symptoms can come on suddenly and clear up on their own within a few days. If it lasts longer than a week, consult a doctor, as it can cause dehydration.

Treating Montezuma's Revenge

When acute diarrhea strikes, most people reach for that bottle of imodium. While imodium will give you temporary relief, if your diet is bad, your symptoms will return. In LGS, diarrhea often occurs when the disease-causing bacteria overwhelm the beneficial bacteria in your system, creating inflammation and leaking of your gut membranes. If this is the case, you need to restore the proper bacterial balance in the bowel by supplying your intestinal tract with more good bacteria. This can be done with probiotics such as *Lactobacillus rhamnosus*, *Lactobacillus acidophilus*, and bifidobacteria found in certain cultured products or in pill or powder form.

Saccharomyces boulardii (*S. boulardii*) is yeast that works to restore your gut function. *S. boulardii* can be most effective for antibiotic-associated diarrhea. It can also provide relief for traveler's diarrhea. Studies suggest it might help your intestines fight off unwanted pathogens and ensure they're absorbing nutrients properly. However, it should be used with caution in people with compromised immune systems.[4]

Causes of Diarrhea

Diarrhea is commonly caused by inflammation of the gastro-intestinal tract. Acute diarrhea, however, might also be produced by bacteria, such as Salmonella and *Clostridium difficile* (*C. difficile*). *C. difficile* is sometimes found in water, eggs, and poultry and can infect the colon and be potentially fatal. Travelers can also experience acute diarrhea when exposed to *Escherichia coli* (*E. coli*), which releases enterotoxins in the gut. It can also be caused by viruses, alcohol, drugs, anxiety, and antibiotics.

There are more than three million cases of diarrhea per year in the United States, and approximately 1 percent to 4 percent of patients with *C. difficile* die from the illness. Children are especially vulnerable to dehydration. We are seeing such a dramatic increase in *C. difficile* infections due to the overuse of powerful antacid medications, which block the stomach's natural ability to kill infectious organisms by producing stomach acid.

Alcohol, milk, soda, and other carbonated or caffeinated drinks might make symptoms worse. Fried and greasy foods, as well as dairy products, are also are also common culprits. If you have diarrhea, stay away from fruits and vegetables that can cause gas, such as

- broccoli
- beans
- peas
- corn
- prunes
- chickpeas
- peppers

As I mentioned previously, *C. difficile* is a potentially serious bacterial disease that can lead to intestinal conditions such as colitis. You might get *C. difficile* disease if you have an illness that requires prolonged use of antibiotics. The disease can also be spread in the hospital, and the elderly are particularly at risk. Taking acid-blocking medications increases your risk of getting a *C. difficile* infection.

Symptoms include the following:

- abdominal pain or tenderness
- fever
- loss of appetite
- nausea
- watery diarrhea (at least three bowel movements per day for two or more days)

Fecal Microbiota Transplants for C. difficile

Fecal microbiota transplants (FMT) have a high "yuck" factor, but they also have a high success rate. If you are diagnosed with *C. difficile*, you might want to consider a fecal transplant because (a) you are feeling miserable, (b) antibiotic treatments have failed, and (c) it can be life-saving. FMT can help people with stubborn, unhealthy gut flora. Patients who have tried long-term antibiotics, or in some cases, probiotics, to no avail—because these treatments do not always work with stubborn *C. difficile* infections—are candidates for FMT. While antibiotics will clear up the infection temporarily, the *C. difficile* keeps coming back. Antibiotics often strip the gut of the good bacteria along with the bad, which makes it difficult for the body to keep *C. difficile* at bay.

How FMT Works

A fecal microbiota transplant works by giving the recipient a boost of healthy bacteria to regenerate his or her own gut flora. This strengthens the person's gut against future infections and stops *C. difficile* from returning.[5]

Hydrochloric Acid Deficiency

Conventional doctors are quick to prescribe antacids to inhibit the production of stomach acid. My experience has shown, however, that most conventional doctors don't have a clue about the risks of having low stomach acid. Often the stomach does not produce enough hydrochloric acid, which is called achlorhydria. This is especially common in older people who are prone to thyroid problems and autoimmune disorders. As you now know, without enough hydrochloric acid, you can't digest the food, which creates abnormal yeast and bacterial overgrowth that cause the tight junctions in the gut to separate and absorb unwanted food particles. Low stomach acid production causes many of the symptoms outlined earlier, including food allergies, bloating, indigestion, constipation, diarrhea, and GERD.

If you think you might have GERD, ask your doctor to measure the pH (acidity) of your stomach by taking what's called the Heidelberg test. The Heidelberg test involves swallowing a pill that is attached to a string. After the pill enters the middle of the stomach, you drink different substances to stimulate hydrochloric production. The pill contains a transducer that sends a signal about the pH of the stomach, which can then be measured.

My Dad's Story

You might recall in the introduction that my father, Ellis Brownstein, was overweight, smoked cigarettes, and had many stomach complaints. After numerous scopes, gastroenterologists diagnosed him with GERD and IBS. He was put on Zantac, the antacid, for life. (This was before the advent of more potent proton-pump inhibitors [PPIs] like Prilosec and Nexium.) It didn't help. Even though my father was taking all the antacid medications, including Tums, he was still suffering from bloating and IBS. When I bought a Heidelberg machine for my practice, my dad was the first patient I used it on to measure his stomach acid production. I found that he wasn't producing enough stomach acid.

I put him on 600 mg of stomach acid pills with every meal, and the results were astounding. After taking the first hydrochloric acid pill, my dad noticed an immediate improvement. "It was miraculous! I felt better—no bloating and no pain," he says. From that moment on, he could eat without discomfort. A few months later, he went back to his gastroenterologist to tell him what he was doing. The physician firmly told my father that he was mistaken: "Ellis, you have too much stomach acid, not too little."

"How do you know I have too much stomach acid?" my father asked. "Did you measure it?"

The doctor paused and then said, "No, I just know it."

My father explained that his primary doctor (me) did a Heidelberg test that showed low stomach acid production. "I am feeling so much better taking a stomach acid pill, and I was feeling awful with the antacid pill," my dad told the specialist. "Why would I go back and take an antacid pill?" The doctor insisted that he needed to take the antacid pill. At that point, my father walked out of that office and never returned. My dad continued taking a hydrochloric acid pill with each meal until he passed away.

Symptoms of Low Stomach Acid
- acne
- bloating, belching, and flatulence immediately after meals
- chronic candida
- feeling full too quickly
- heartburn (often thought to be caused by too much stomach acid)
- indigestion, diarrhea, or constipation
- rectal itching
- undigested food in stools

Treatment for Acid Deficiency
People with achlorhydria, including those taking PPIs, need to have their vitamin B12 levels evaluated and treated with vitamin B12 injections when indicated. Injectable forms of vitamin

B12 have proven to be extremely effective. Keep in mind, however, that oral B12 supplements that you buy at your local drugstore or health food store will not be absorbed well when there is not enough acid in the stomach. Likewise, oral, nasal, and sublingual (taken on the tongue) forms are not as effective as injectable B12.

A proven treatment (and the one I prescribed for my father) for low stomach acid is taking stomach acid (hydrochloric) pills with each meal. The bloating and LGS goes away almost immediately. It is one of the most satisfying treatments I employ. Typically I prescribe between 60 mg and 600 mg. It's taken at the beginning of the meals and never on an empty stomach. The only side effect of taking stomach acid pills is that they can sometimes cause burning. If taken at the beginning of a meal, however, these adverse reactions rarely occur. If there is burning, I suggest stopping the stomach acid supplement. Elderly patients might have to be on the pills for life (again, like my dad), but younger patients might be able to correct on their own with nutritional balancing only.

Table 1: Conditions That Might Cause Achlorhydria

Autoimmune thyroid diseases such as Hashimoto's disease

H. pylori **infection** (see page 62)

Long-term use of PPIs (e.g., Nexium and Prilosec) and other antacid drugs

Mucolipidosis type IV, an inherited disorder characterized by delayed development and vision impairment that worsens over time[6]

Pernicious anemia, a decrease in red blood cells that occurs when the intestines cannot properly absorb vitamin B12[7]

Gastritis

Simply put, gastritis is inflammation of the stomach lining. As I explained earlier, the stomach's job in the digestive process is to acidify its contents so the food can be broken down, and the stomach excretes a lining of mucous (gastric mucosa) to protect itself from the acid. Some people don't produce enough mucus, which inflames and irritates the stomach. If gastritis is severe enough or left untreated, you can get erosions in the stomach wall that will cause ulcers and, in some cases, increase your risk of stomach cancer.

Causes of Gastritis

Gastritis can be caused by irritation due to excessive alcohol use, chronic vomiting, stress, or the use of certain medications such as aspirin or other anti-inflammatory drugs. It can also be caused by the following:

- **Bile reflux**. This is a backflow of bile into the stomach coming from the bile tract that connects to the liver and gallbladder.
- *Helicobacter pylori*. *H. pylori* is a bacterium that lives in the mucous lining of the stomach.
- **Infections**. These can be caused by bacteria and viruses.

Symptoms of Gastritis

Symptoms of gastritis vary depending on the individual, and for some people, there are no symptoms. The most common symptoms include

- abdominal bloating
- abdominal pain

- black stools
- burning or gnawing feeling in the stomach between meals or at night
- hiccups
- indigestion
- loss of appetite
- nausea or recurrent upset stomach
- vomiting

How Is Gastritis Diagnosed?

To diagnose gastritis, your doctor will review your medical history and perform a thorough physical evaluation. He or she might recommend an upper endoscopy (a.k.a. scope) to look at your stomach lining, blood tests to screen for *H. pylori* infection and anemia, and a stool test.

Treatments for Gastritis

People with gastritis often take antacids such as Maalox and Mylanta or H2 blockers, including Prilosec and Nexium, to control stomach acid. These conventional treatments are only approved for a few weeks, and the long-term use of these medications is fraught with adverse effects. Preferred therapies include the following:

Note: Once the underlying cause disappears, the gastritis usually does too.

- **Using antibiotics/acid blockers** plus an acid-blocking drug (used for heartburn) for gastritis caused by *H. pylori* infection
- **Getting B12 vitamin shots** for gastritis caused by "pernicious" anemia

- **Eliminating irritants** from your diet, such as dairy or gluten, and avoiding spicy foods
- **Taking supplements** such as zinc and magnesium that your stomach needs to produce a healthy mucous coating

H. pylori Infection

H. pylori is a spiral-shaped bacterium that is found in the inner surface of the stomach. Approximately two-thirds of the world's population is infected in *H. pylori*, which is the cause of most ulcers. It occurs in approximately 20 percent of people younger than forty and 50 percent of those age sixty or older. It can be diagnosed with a blood test, biopsy, or breath test. Many factors contribute to this infection, including a poor diet high in refined foods—especially refined sugars—which weakens the immune system and decreases the body's ability to fight off these infections.

However, the number-one factor I see in my practice that triggers *H. pylori* infection is low stomach acid production (achlorhydria), resulting in an elevated stomach pH. If the pH of the stomach is in the normal range (pH 1–3), my experience has shown that *H. pylori* infections are rare. When there is inadequate production of hydrochloric acid, they are much more common.

Treatments for H. pylori *Infection*

Conventional treatment for *H. pylori* involves PPIs and antibiotics. Unfortunately, antibiotics not only kill bad bacteria such as *H. pylori* but also harm the good intestinal bacteria such a *L. acidophilus*. Prescribing antibiotics at these high rates can also create bacteria that are resistant to modern medications, which

The *H. pylori* Breath Test

H. pylori produces an enzyme called urease, which breaks urea down into ammonia and carbon dioxide. During the test, a tablet containing urea (a chemical made of nitrogen and a minimally radioactive carbon) is swallowed and the amount of exhaled carbon dioxide is measured. This indicates the presence of *H. pylori* in the stomach.

can have a devastating effect on public health. The following are my preferred treatments:

- **Acid supplements**. If the pH of the stomach is too high, one to ten grains (60–600 mg) of hydrochloric acid supplements with meals will often resolve the condition. If one experiences excess burning with hydrochloric acid supplements, it should not be taken. Those with ulcers in the gastric lining should not take these supplements until they are healed. If there is *H. pylori* infection, follow my other recommendations for two weeks before beginning the acid supplements.
- **Dietary changes**. The first and best step in any successful *H. pylori* treatment is eliminating refined foods, especially sugar. I've observed dramatic improvements in my patients who have done this.
- **Mastic**. In addition to maintaining adequate pH of the stomach, I recommend taking the herbal supplement mastic, which can be taken in tablet form or

chewed as gum. Mastic is produced by a shrub native to the Mediterranean region and contains the active ingredients that are effective for eliminating *H. pylori*. A study published in *New England Journal of Medicine* in 1998 confirmed the efficacy of mastic in treating *H. pylori* infections. Not only is mastic less expensive than the recommended regimen of FDA-approved antibiotics and acid blockers; there are fewer adverse side effects (although some patients have experienced upset stomach).

- **Oregano oil**. Oregano oil has helped many of my patients overcome *H. pylori*. My experience has shown that 50 mg of oregano oil (sustained release works the best) three times daily, with meals, is consistently effective.[8]

Peptic Ulcers

This common condition caused by the breakdown of the stomach lining can lead to bleeding. This can be painful even without food in the stomach and is sometimes relieved after taking an antacid.

What Causes Ulcers?

Ulcers are caused by *H. pylori* overgrowth, nutrient deficiencies, and a poor diet. Ulcers can also be caused by the overuse of painkillers, such as aspirin, and nonsteroidal anti-inflammatories, such as ibuprofen or naproxen.

Flavonoids

Research suggests that flavonoids, also known as bioflavonoids, might be an effective treatment for stomach ulcers. Flavonoids are compounds that occur naturally in many fruits and vegetables. Foods and drinks that contain flavonoids include

- apples
- berries
- broccoli
- kale
- legumes
- red grapes
- teas (especially green tea)

Caveat: Citrus fruits and red wines, which are also rich in flavonoids, can irritate a stomach ulcer.

Flavonoids are referred to as "gastroprotective," which means that they defend the lining of the stomach and could allow ulcers to heal. According to the Linus Pauling Institute, there are no side effects of consuming flavonoids in the amount found in a typical diet, but higher amounts of flavonoids might interfere with blood clotting. The best way to get flavonoids is through foods, but you can also take them as supplements.

Licorice (Deglycyrrhizinated)

Don't worry about wrapping your head or mouth around that second unpronounceable word in this heading. *Deglycyrrhizinated* is the technical term for licorice that has had the sweetness extracted, so I'm not talking about Twizzlers here. One study showed that deglycyrrhizinated licorice might help ulcers heal by inhibiting the growth of *H. pylori*. Deglycyrrhiz-

Caveat: Eating more than 2 ounces daily for more than two weeks can make existing heart problems or high blood pressure worse.[9]

inated licorice is available as a supplement. I have used this many times over the years with very good success. Licorice works by coating breaks in the mucosal lining of the stomach and esophagus allowing the body time to heal the lesions.

Probiotics

Probiotics found in fermented foods or supplements have been shown to destroy the offending *H. pylori* that causes ulcers and improve the recovery rate for patients with ulcers.

Garlic

Garlic extract has been shown to inhibit *H. pylori* growth in lab, animal, and human trials. If you don't like the taste or smell of garlic, you can take garlic extract supplements. Garlic acts as a blood thinner, so ask your doctor before taking it if you use prescription blood thinners.[10]

Antioxidants

A vitamin-rich diet can help your body heal ulcers. Foods containing polyphenol, a type of antioxidant, can protect you from ulcers and help ulcers heal. Polyphenol-rich foods and seasonings include

- black olives
- blueberries
- dark chocolate
- dried rosemary
- Mexican oregano[11]

What to Avoid

Greasy and acidic foods are most likely to irritate your stomach, as are spicy foods. To reduce ulcer pain, avoid

- carbonated beverages
- chilies and hot peppers
- coffee, including decaf
- deep fried foods

- processed foods
- refined salty red meats

Mindful Eating

If you're like most people, you think more about eating foods than about

> **Caveat**: It is a wives' tale that stress causes ulcers. Stress can exacerbate the condition, but it won't create it.

"digesting" them. Even if you are eating a healthy diet full of berries, greens, and unprocessed foods, your body needs to break down and absorb these foods in order to get the full nutritional benefits. But problems such as stress, poor dietary choices, food sensitivities, and other factors can disrupt this process, preventing you from getting all the nutrients you need. That's why making a few changes in how you eat can give you more energy, help you lose excess weight, reduce your feeling of being bloated, and regulate your trips to the bathroom. The following are some tips for mindful eating that will optimize your health by altering some of your unhealthy habits.

Chew Your Food Thoroughly

Unlike Europeans, for whom meals are a time to relax, gather with friends and family, and savor food, Americans often eat on the run. Food vendors that sell their wares on the street encourage people to eat and walk, which is not the way we are meant to ingest our meals. If you're the first person to clean your plate, chances are you are not chewing thoroughly. Taking small bites and chewing breaks down food and activates enzymes in your mouth that aid digestion. In fact, studies from Purdue University found that people who chewed almonds (a superfood) forty times absorbed more healthy fat than when they chewed them just ten times. The reason, according to Richard D. Mattes, PhD, the author of this study, is that chewing breaks down the cell walls of the foods we eat, making them easier to digest. If you don't want to count bites, just wait until the food is mushy before swallowing.

Take Time to Enjoy Your Food

If you are stressed after a long day or you're thinking about work or problems at home during your lunch break, your brain will release a stress hormone called cortisol that will make your heart beat faster and give you a rush of adrenaline. This process is the remnant of a natural animal instinct called "fight or flight." Adrenaline was useful for our ancestors when they came face-to-face with danger, such as a saber-toothed tiger; however, this hormonal reaction can wreak havoc on our digestive system, which slows down or stops so our bodies can channel energy into dealing with the stress.

Similarly, multitasking (reading, texting, talking on the phone) while eating can interfere with your body's absorption of nutrients. Try to relax as much as possible during meals and savor every bite. And besides kick-starting the digestive process, chewing stimulates our taste buds. Not only will your stomach be happier; you will enjoy your food so much more!

The Four Rs for Healthy Digestion

A simple way to remember my recommendations for recognizing and treating LGS are the four *R*s for healthy digestion:

Remove. Clean up your diet by getting rid of the bad stuff causing inflammation in your gut (and elsewhere), including refined sugars, flour, soda, and processed foods.

Replace. Replace healthy flora through probiotics and gut-healthy foods and beverages.

Reinocculate. Build up your gut with the right nutrients, supplements, and other therapies that bring down inflammation.

Repair. By doing the three steps above, your leaky gut and digestive system will eventually repair itself!

Next, learn how LGS can cause achy muscles and joints, including arthritic conditions, and what you can do to treat them.

Heal Your Achy Muscles and Joints

I've had thirty-six orthopedic operations, had two fused
ankles, my knees, hands and wrists don't work . . .
other than that, everything is great.

—Bill Walton, former NBA All-Star basketball player

My patients come to me with a variety of conditions, including arthritis, fibromyalgia, osteoporosis, and chronic fatigue syndrome (CFS), all of which can be brought on or made worse by leaky gut syndrome (LGS). Most go first to conventional doctors, who prescribe medications that have no benefits, leaving them desperate for something to improve their condition and get back to a healthy life. Luckily, there are ways to treat these conditions without using drugs that will make you either sicker or more exhausted. In fact, there is not a single prescription drug therapy that treats the underlying cause of any of the conditions mentioned previously. The following are the most common muscle and joint disorders, along with holistic treatments and therapies that I have used to successfully treat them.

Arthritis

Arthritis, which is an inflammation of the joints and the tissue around them, is one of the most prevalent conditions in medicine today, affecting thirty-two million Americans (nearly one in eight people). It is estimated that by the year 2020, sixty million Americans will be suffering from arthritis as the population ages. It is broad term that can accompany many different diseases, including rheumatoid arthritis and osteoarthritis (sometimes called degenerative joint disease, or "wear and tear" arthritis).

The connection between LGS and these conditions is the leaky membrane that allows foreign proteins and bacteria to enter the bloodstream, which creates inflammation. Chronic inflammation can cause nearly any arthritic illness, and when the inflammation is revved up, it can exacerbate flare-ups. Let's say you have arthritis in your knee, for example. If you're eating badly, you will get an inflamed, leaky gut, which leads to gut contents gaining access to the bloodstream. This can cause inflammation and, if your knee is your weak point, make your arthritic knee worse. After more than one hundred years of relying on drugs and imaging tests to diagnose and treat arthritis, conventional doctors still do not know what causes arthritis. Unbelievably, in most cases, traditional medical approaches do not even search for the underlying cause. This begs the question: If you don't understand the cause of an illness, then how can you effectively treat it? I'll tell you how.

What Causes Arthritis?

Based on my clinical experience and research dating back more than a century, I've found that arthritis is caused by infectious agents, such as bacteria, viruses, parasites, and yeast. Patients with these kinds of infections will frequently respond well (often dramatically well) to appropriate antibiotic therapy. There are numerous bacteria, viruses, and fungi that have been implicated in various forms of arthritis (see Table 1), but a bacteria known as mycoplasma is suspected to be one of main causative factors. Mycoplasma was first isolated in humans by Dr. Louis Dienes in 1932, followed by Dr. Albert Sabin, who was able to isolate mycoplasma in arthritic mice in 1938.

Table 1: Infectious Causes of Arthritis

candida

chlamydia

Coxiella

Brucella

Borrelia burgdorferi

fungi

hepatitis B

HIV

Mycobacterium tuberculosis

mycoplasma

Neisseria

parvovirus B19

rickettsia

Staphylococcus aureus

Streptococcus

Treponema pallidum

Treatments for Arthritis

This lack of understanding by traditional medicine has led to treatments that are not only ineffective but often toxic. The most commonly used treatment for arthritic conditions has been nonsteroidal anti-inflammatory drugs (NSAIDs), which have been used for more than sixty years. When these drugs fail, as they often do, more powerful steroids such as chemotherapeutic agents are prescribed. If those fail, drugs that drastically inhibit the immune system's ability to fight infections are utilized. In my experience, these kinds of drug therapies have been a failure of epic proportions. While these medications might temporarily alleviate the symptoms of arthritis, they do little to reverse or even halt the progression of the illness. Additionally, NSAIDs do not provide the body with the substances needed to heal it. In fact, the toxicity of these drugs will inhibit the body's ability to heal and even weaken the immune system, making it more susceptible to illnesses. Research has consistently shown that long-term NSAID use is associated with poor outcomes in arthritic patients.

One frightening statistic estimates that the use of NSAIDs can be fatal, with 16,500 rheumatoid arthritis or osteoarthritis patients dying annually due to toxic side effects. Further studies have shown that the prolonged use of NSAIDs will inhibit cartilage formation in arthritic patients and actually worsen the condition.

In contrast, the holistic approach to treating arthritis is to search for an underlying cause and then develop a program that addresses that cause. Arthritis is not caused by a deficiency of NSAIDs. A holistic approach uses a combination of safe, natural therapies, with or without drugs (small doses of antibiotics might be necessary to treat the infections listed in Table 1), that target the underlying cause while supporting the body's immune system as it recovers. Treating arthritis, and the other conditions in this chapter and throughout the book, requires a regimen of vitamins, minerals, natural hormones, and water, as well as a balanced diet and detoxification of the body.

If you want an additional supplement for your joint pain, try Limbex, which I prescribe to patients in my practice. Limbex is a clinically tested dietary supplement formulated to promote healthy joints and connective tissue. There are eleven natural ingredients, including glucosamine, chondroitin sulfate, turmeric root extract, and a Boswellia extract called ApresFlex.

I believe the best results are achieved when these therapies are used in combination, rather than individually.[1]

Patti's Story

Patti was a forty-one-year-old woman who came to me in a wheelchair. She had severe rheumatoid arthritis in her knees and other joints that prevented her from walking. An avid cyclist, she told me her goals were to walk and ride a bike again. "I got up for work one day and my thumb was very sore," she told me during her medical history. "I thought I just slept on it wrong. This went away after a few weeks, but then my arm started hurting. The pain didn't stop for days, and then a different joint would start hurting. After the birth of my son eight years ago, the pain and fatigue intensified. My hands were so swollen I had trouble changing my baby's diapers."

Upon examination, I could see that in addition to her knees, her wrists and knuckles were twice their normal size, and they were red and warm (a sign of inflammation). She looked and felt miserable. Patti saw several rheumatologists who prescribed chemotherapy drugs that made her so sick, she felt like the drugs were killing her. Her doctor also put her on high-dose anti-inflammatory medications, which gave her some relief but caused stomach distress.

I did my usual dietary history and found that she wasn't drinking enough water in addition to eating a high-carbohydrate diet that consisted of too many refined foods such as pasta and bread. She ate some organic fruits and vegetables, but not enough, and her stomach was bloated and tender—the exact symptoms of LGS. For someone like Patti, I look for bacterial and viral infections like mycoplasma and chlamydia, which are common in arthritis patients. I took some fluid from her knee and sent it to the lab. I also ordered a stool analysis from a specialized lab to look for an imbalance in her gut flora.

I told Patti to start drinking more water and to eat more whole foods. She would also need to eliminate the pasta and grains from her diet and replace them with proteins free of hormones and pesticides. When she came back in three weeks, she wasn't feeling much better, but her stomach wasn't bloated or giving her pain. The laboratory results revealed that Patti was suffering from an active infection of *Mycoplasma pneumoniae*, a bacterium that can cause lung infections as well as joint problems. She also had low levels of healthy gut bacteria such as *L. acidophilus*.

I treated Patti with a low-dose antibiotic of doxycycline three days a week. Her blood tests also revealed a hypothyroid (underactive thyroid) condition, as well as low iodine, vitamin C, and magnesium levels. I put her on a natural thyroid supplement as well as a probiotic and a prebiotic to counteract the antibiotics she was taking as well as to replenish her gut with healthy bacteria. She was also dairy and gluten intolerant, so she immediately went on a gluten-, dairy-, and grain-free diet.

The results of this treatment were nothing short of spectacular. When I saw her again in six weeks, she was out of the wheelchair and using a walker. I remember smiling when I saw her walk into the office. The swelling, warmth, and redness of her joints were down, and she was feeling markedly better. She reported that whenever she went off her new diet, her body and gut would get inflamed again, so she promised to stick to the program from then on. The next time she saw me, she was walking with a cane. She continued the therapy, and within a year, she came back to see me with a video of her and her husband riding a tandem bike! The video brought tears to my eyes.

Fibromyalgia

Fibromyalgia is chronic arthritis-related condition with symptoms that can include widespread musculoskeletal pain, fatigue, depression, headaches, mental fogginess, and bowel and bladder problems. A type of central-pain syndrome, fibromyalgia is believed to be the result of a problem in the way the brain processes pain signals. I find that many of my patients who have arthritis also have many of the signs and symptoms of fibromyalgia. People with this condition can find it debilitating, and more women get it than men, making up 90 percent of the cases diagnosed, according to US government statistics. Men get the disorder too, but they tend to get fewer and milder symptoms than women. The reason for this gender difference isn't completely understood, but some believe it has to do with hormones produced during the reproductive years, as women find the pain is more severe during their periods.

Incredibly, some conventional doctors don't believe this disorder is real, which can be extremely frustrating for patients who have it.

Causes of Fibromyalgia

Fibromyalgia can have different causes, including bacterial infections, viral infections, or nutrient and hormonal imbalances, such as low thyroid, estrogen, testosterone, or cortisol levels, so the treatments differ depending on the individual's root problem. A comprehensive hormonal analysis should be undertaken for all fibromyalgia patients.

Fibromyalgia Treatments

The most common triggers for fibromyalgia are simple sugars and refined foods that lack basic vitamins and minerals. Because our bodies need to absorb vitamins and minerals in order to maintain healthy immune and digestive systems, when we are nutritionally deficient—sometimes caused by LGS—it is difficult for these systems to function optimally. If this continues, we are prone to infections that target injured areas of your body. This becomes a downward spiral in health.

The first step in treating fibromyalgia is to stop eating refined foods that deplete vital nutrients and to supply the body with the right nutrients so it can function properly. A good general treatment for fibromyalgia is to go on a low glycemic, gluten-free diet, as follows:

- no gluten
- no refined oil
- no refined salt
- no refined sugar

Gluten and Inflammation

It is now widely accepted that gluten, a protein found in wheat, rye, and barley, can play a part in a host of ailments, including digestive problems, fatigue, headache, skin rash, and possibly fibromyalgia as well as other chronic conditions like arthritis. Gluten can trigger damaging inflammation in the small intestines, which can cause serious reactions in people with celiac disease, a serious autoimmune disorder that we will discuss in Chapter 4. The good news is that most supermarkets today offer an array of gluten-free products for those who are sensitive or allergic to this protein.

Spanish researchers who were curious about whether gluten contributed to fibromyalgia conducted a study that was published in a 2014 issue of *Rheumatology International*. They examined twenty patients who had fibromyalgia for gluten sensitivity while not fully meeting the criteria for celiac disease. After going on a gluten-free diet for sixteen months, all patients reported improvement in the level of widespread chronic pain, fatigue, gastrointestinal symptoms, migraine, and depression. "This report shows that remarkable clinical improvement can be achieved with a gluten-free diet in patients with [fibromyalgia], even if celiac disease has been ruled out," the study's authors wrote.

Another larger study published that same year in *Arthritis Research and Therapy* evaluated the one-year effect of a gluten-free diet in ninety-seven women with both fibromyalgia and irritable bowel syndrome (IBS). Similarly, none of the women were diagnosed with celiac disease. However, fifty-eight participants tested positive for inflammation of the small intestine (frequently found in people with LGS, food allergies, autoimmune disorders, bacterial infections, and those taking NSAIDs). The gluten-free diet produced a significant improvement in symptoms of both the IBS and the fibromyalgia groups.

The Importance of Hormones

Hormones are the chemical substances produced from glands that control nearly every physiological reaction in the body.

Every single muscle, organ, and cell depend on adequate thyroid hormone levels, so the importance of hormones for optimal functioning cannot be overstated.

I have found that even a slight thyroid hormone deficiency (hypothyroidism) can have a tremendous impact on overall health. In fact, it's nearly impossible for individuals with any chronic disorder to overcome their illness without treating their hormone imbalances.

Patients with fibromyalgia and arthritis are particularly susceptible. The conventional treatment for hypothyroidism is to put a patient on a synthetic hormone such as Synthroid. There are other natural thyroid replacement alternatives, however, that are safer and more effective. The medical reasons for this are complex, but suffice it to say that common sense might tell you that using hormones that are similar to the ones naturally produced in your system would be a better choice.

In contrast, I have found the natural thyroid hormone, known as Armour Thyroid, to be far more effective in treating these conditions.

Studies Reveal Food Additives Can Cause Fibromyalgia Symptoms

For years, researchers have suspected that food additives (called excitotoxins) might worsen fibromyalgia symptoms in some people. Excitotoxins include three amino acids: glutamate, aspartate, and L-cysteine, which are commonly used as flavor enhancers and sugar substitutes. Some of the earliest evidence of a fibromyalgia-excitotoxin connection was seen in a 2001 case study published in *Annals of Pharmacotherapy*. Four people with fibromyalgia who did not respond well to other treatments became totally or nearly symptom-free within months of removing monosodium glutamate (MSG) or aspartame

Table 2: Symptoms of Hypothyroidism

The symptoms of hypothyroidism include	
arthritis	headaches and migraines
brittle nails	heart disease
cold extremities/cold intolerance	hypercholesteremia
constipation	hypoglycemia
depression	infertility
difficulty getting up in the morning	poor memory
diminished sweating	menstrual disorders/ premenstrual syndrome
dry skin, acne, psoriasis, eczema	ovarian cysts
fatigue and weakness	obesity/difficulty losing weight
fibrocystic breast disease	recurrent infections

from their diets. All had symptoms return after MSG was reintroduced.

In another study published in 2012 in *Clinical and Experimental Rheumatology*, fifty-seven patients with fibromyalgia and IBS symptoms were put on a diet without MSG and aspartame. After four weeks on the elimination diet, 84 percent of those completing the diet reported that their symptoms improved by more than 30 percent. Adding MSG back into the diet resulted in a significant return of symptoms. While there have been some conflicting results in other studies, it is wise to err on the side of caution if you have fibromyalgia symptoms by avoiding these additives.

Vitamin D

Vitamin D is necessary for maintaining the structural integrity of bones and teeth and for maintaining a healthy hormonal system. Many fibromyalgia and arthritis patients have low levels of vitamin D. We need vitamin D to absorb calcium, and our bodies produce it when our skin is directly exposed to the sun. Research has shown a connection between low levels of vitamin D and arthritis, osteoporosis, chronic widespread musculoskeletal pain, high blood pressure, and autoimmune diseases.

While it is not known for sure whether vitamin D supplements help relieve pain or other symptoms of fibromyalgia in people who are deficient, an Austrian study published in 2014 in the journal *Pain* suggests that it might. Thirty women with fibromyalgia and low blood levels of vitamin D received either a vitamin D supplement or a placebo. The treatment group experienced improvement in physical functioning, morning fatigue, and pain, while the placebo group was unchanged.

Although the data presented in the study are promising, study author Florian Wepner, MD, an orthopedist at Vienna's Orthopedic Hospital Speising, notes that more studies are needed to better determine the potential role of vitamin D in fibromyalgia treatment. In the meantime, I believe that vitamin D is a safe supplement that can be used along with certain medications and other nondrug treatments for fibromyalgia and arthritis. The recommended dose is 1,000–2,000 units per day. Note: Your vitamin levels should be checked periodically.[2]

"SHINE" Treatment Found to Help with Fibromyalgia
Jacob Teitelbaum, MD, director of the Practitioners Alliance Network and author of *From Fatigued to Fantastic*, not only

treats patients with fibromyalgia and CFS; he has had both conditions since 1975. He offers a clinically tested protocol called SHINE (sleep, hormonal deficiencies, infections, nutritional supplementation, and exercise), which I also recommend to my patients.

1. **Sleep**. In order to get well and be pain-free, it is critical to get eight to nine hours of sleep each night. I recommend starting with natural therapies and supplements such as melatonin and valerian.

2. **Hormonal deficiencies**. The hypothalamus is the main control center, via the pituitary, for most of the glands in the body. Most of the normal ranges for blood tests were not developed to detect hypothalamic suppression common to these syndromes. Because of this (and for a number of other reasons), it is usually necessary to treat fibromyalgia with natural thyroid, adrenal, and ovarian and testicular hormones, even if your blood tests come back normal. These hormones have been found to be reasonably safe when used in low doses. Low thyroid—which results in fatigue, weight gain, cold intolerance, and even unexplained infertility—is especially common, and the majority of those who benefit from a natural thyroid supplement have normal lab tests, so a treatment trial should be given using natural thyroid hormones if you are symptomatic.

3. **Infections**. Many studies have shown immune system dysfunction in patients who have fibromyalgia and CFS, which can result in many unusual infections (such as the ones listed in Table 1), including parasites

and other bowel infections, antibiotic sensitive infections, and most importantly, fungal/candida infections.

4. **Nutritional supplementation**. Widespread nutritional deficiencies are common and require dozens of nutritional supplements, including a good daily multivitamin and ribose, which can jumpstart your energy level. In Dr. Teitelbaum's initial study, ribose was found to increase energy levels an average of 45 percent in just three weeks. A second study conducted by eighty-one physicians (currently being prepared for publication) showed an average of more than a 59 percent increase in energy in those with CFS and fibromyalgia.

5. **Exercise as tolerated**. I realize that exercising is difficult for many people, especially those with aches, pains, and fatigue, but movement is just what the doctor ordered. Do not push to the point of crashing the next day. Start by walking as long as you comfortably can (even if that is only two minutes). After ten weeks on a treatment (or sooner, if you are up to it), start to increase your walks by up to one minute more each day until you reach an hour of walking. After that, you can increase your intensity level.

Rachel's Story

Rachel, a fifty-two-year-old businesswoman, came to see me complaining that she had no energy and that she was achy all over. "I was fine until five years ago," she explained. "I woke up one day aching. I thought I had the flu, but the pains never went away. Along with aching, I am always tired. I get no answers from any of the doctors I've seen. Some even told me it's in my head, but this is real!"

She saw numerous health care practitioners, some of whom suggested antidepressants that didn't help her. After years without relief, she felt like there was nowhere to turn. "I don't want to live like this!" she told me as she wept in my office. "Why won't the doctors believe me? I am not making this up—I hurt all over." Rachel's fatigue and muscle achiness got to the point where she was no longer able to exercise, a heavy blow for someone who was once quite physically active. Even worse was the fact that she could barely get through the work day or take care of her family when she got home.

I gave Rachel a physical, including a blood work-up and dietary history. When I asked her how she felt when she exerted herself, she said, "If I try to do anything beyond everyday activities, I'm in bed for two or three days, so I try to pace myself."

A dietary history revealed that she was eating fast food and drinking four cups of coffee a day, with not much water. She was also eating lots of candy to give her temporary boosts of energy. She frequently felt bloated after meals, and her stomach hurt her as soon as she started eating in the mornings, and the pain would persist throughout the day. "I read an article about leaky gut syndrome, and it sounds like I might have the symptoms. Is that what's wrong with me, Dr. Brownstein? What should I do about it? Please, help me!" she said.

I suspected that she was right about the LGS, and I talked to her about eliminating all refined foods, sugars, and grains that get turned quickly into sugar. Instead, I advised her to eat a whole-food diet with lots of fruits and vegetables and good sources of protein free of hormones and pesticides. I also had her drink two liters of water a day. I asked to see her again in three weeks to go over her test results. When she came back, she wasn't as tired or achy, although she still felt a bit fatigued. She had some bloating issues, especially after she ate sugar. But she finally had a glimmer of hope that things could be better for her.

Her blood tests showed that she was low in vitamin B1 (thiamine) and low in iodine and iron. Her thyroid hormones were also in the lower level of the range, making her hypothyroid. I corrected her nutritional deficiencies by giving her 50.0 mg of thiamine and 12.5 mg of iodine daily, and I told her I'd recheck her levels in six weeks.

When she returned, she said she felt like a new person. Her stomach wasn't hurting her anymore, her energy level was back, and her mood was better. I retested her thyroid levels, which had increased thanks to the iodine supplement. At that point, she felt about 80 to 90 percent better and had more energy and almost no achiness.

At a recent office visit, Rachel said to me, "I just want to thank you. Out of all the doctors I saw, you were the only doctor who asked me about my diet! Even when I asked if my condition had anything to do with what I was eating, they said no. It wasn't easy, but I cleaned up my diet like you told me to, and all my stomach problems went away. I feel like I have a whole new body! Now if I cheat on my diet, I begin to feel the old symptoms again. I don't ever want to feel like I did before, so that's all the motivation I need to stick with the program."

> **Takeaway**: If the body is supplied with the right food and nutrients, it can do miraculous things. Once you get rid of the inflammatory-provoking foods, the stomach can close up the gaps that let the bad stuff seep in!

Tips for Getting a Good Night's Sleep

There are various ways to fight insomnia and boost your melatonin (the natural sleep hormone) at night, starting with establishing a regular circadian rhythm. Here are some ways to make sure you get the restorative rest you need:

- **Wind down**. Get in the habit of preparing your brain for sleep by winding down activity in the evening and going to bed at the same time every night.
- **Shut off your TV and shut down your devices**. Save your e-mailing and texting for the morning and record your favorite late-night shows to watch earlier in the evening if you want to get to sleep. The high-frequency blue light emitted from these screens will keep you up by keeping your melatonin down.
- **Cover electrical displays**. Our bedrooms are often lit up by tiny lights coming from our alarm clocks, DVRs, phones, and other electrical gadgets. Cover them up before you go to bed and keep the room dark.
- **Use a flashlight**. Don't switch on the light if you have to get up to use the bathroom at night. Use a flashlight instead or get a light dimmer so it's easier to fall back to sleep. (Don't do this if you are not steady on your feet.)
- **Keep out the natural light**. Use heavy curtains or shades to block the light coming through your windows in the morning (or city lights if you are an urban dweller). Consider wearing a sleep mask. The darker the room, the deeper the sleep.
- **Keep the room colder**. When we fall asleep, our bodies naturally cool off. Helping your body get to that lower temperature faster can encourage deeper sleep.[3]

Osteoporosis

Osteoporosis, which means "porous bone," can cause thinning bones and painful fractures. Risk factors for osteoporosis include aging (especially in women), low body weight, menopause, smoking, and some medications. Prevention and treatment include nutritional calcium and vitamin D and exercise, including strength training. When bones become weak, they can more easily break from a fall or, in serious cases, from sneezing, coughing, or minor bumps.

Causes of Osteoporosis
The following are risk factors for developing osteoporosis:

- **Genetics**. Women are more at risk, but anyone of thin build and of Northern European or Asian descent is at higher risk. Studies of mothers and daughters have shown that heredity plays a role in bone density.
- **Menopause**. When women stop menstruating, estrogen levels decrease dramatically. As much as half of a woman's total bone loss occurs within the first ten years following menopause.
- **Not enough calcium**. Calcium intake plays a vital role in bone mineralization during our childhood years and is essential for building strong bones. Likewise, calcium intake continues to be important to slow down bone loss as we age.
- **Lack of vitamin D**. Vitamin D plays a pivotal role in allowing the body to absorb calcium.
- **Inactivity**. Weight-bearing exercises are especially good for increasing bone mass, but walking and

running can also help maintain bone density. The "use it or lose it" rule applies here, so inactive people lose bone density faster than those who are active. Conversely, regular physical activity strengthens both muscles and bones, slows down bone loss, and decreases the risk of injury from falls.

- **Smoking**. The relationship between bone loss and smoking has been confirmed by numerous studies. However, once you quit smoking, even if it's later in life, the bone loss caused by this habit can be minimized.

- **Excessive alcohol**. People who drink alcohol to excess are more prone to fractures. This might be partially due to the diuretic effect of alcohol, which causes calcium depletion through the urine. Alcohol can also decrease the absorption of calcium from the intestines and cause deficiencies in vitamin D and magnesium, both of which are important to bone health.

- **Coffee**. Having more than two cups a day might contribute to accelerated bone loss.

- **High acid-ash diet**. Recent research has suggested that eating an acid-ash producing diet (high in animal protein and grains, low in vegetables and fruit) causes an increase in urinary excretion of calcium, which leads to bone loss.

- **Medications**. Certain medications, such as steroids, antacids, and anticonvulsants, might contribute to demineralization of the bone.

Symptoms of Osteoporosis

How do you know if you might have osteoporosis? A fall that causes a fractured bone or joint is one red flag. Also look out for the following symptoms:

- a gradual loss of height and an accompanying stooped posture
- backache
- fractures of the spine, wrist, or hip (hip fractures are extremely common in elderly patients)

Nancy's Story

A seventy-eight-year-old retired schoolteacher went to her doctor for a routine checkup and was diagnosed with osteoporosis. Her bone density test did, in fact, indicate a loss of bone matter. She was told that she needed to take Fosamax, an osteoporosis medication, for the rest of her life. When she came to me for a second opinion, she said she had been having stomach issues for years, and the osteoporosis drug only made them worse. She would have stomach pains after meals and only felt better when she didn't eat.

She said she wasn't exercising and that she was eating a high-carb, low-protein diet filled with pasta, bread, and cereal. She was also drinking soda and only one or two glasses of water a day. I ordered bloodwork and a stool test, and the lab found that she and low amounts of good bacteria and high levels of candida (a yeast organism). She was also low in vitamin D and vitamin K, both of which the bones need to remineralize, a process that makes them stronger and less likely to break.

I told her to cut out refined foods, to eat whole foods, and to supplement with probiotics, fermented foods, and more water. After four months on this new diet, her stomach pains

> **Note**: If you develop a sudden backache or severe back pain, it could indicate an osteoporosis-related spinal compression fracture. If your dental X-rays show a significant loss of bone in the jaw, consult your doctor immediately.[4]

disappeared. I treated the candida with oregano oil and Citricidal, a natural compound made from the seed and pulp of a grapefruit. I also gave her a probiotic supplement to replenish the good bacteria flora in her gut in addition to the probiotic foods. When I saw her again, all her symptoms had gone away, her gut was better, and she was feeling more energetic. Six months later, another bone density test revealed that her osteoporosis had been reversed.

New Findings Show Calcium Supplements Can Be Bad for Your Heart

Nothing beats calcium for your bones, but a recent study conducted at Johns Hopkins University's School of Medicine in Baltimore has shown that calcium supplements, which used to be the go-to treatment for osteoporosis, are not good for your heart. Researchers analyzed data from 10 years of medical tests on more than 2,700 adults. Participants ranged in age from 45 to 85, and they were questioned on their daily diet and the supplements they took. Participants also underwent CT scans aimed at measuring calcification (hardening) of the arteries, which is a known risk factor

Takeaway: Get your calcium by eating a healthy diet free of refined foods.

of heart disease. The research showed that people who took calcium supplements had a significant increase in the risk of plaque buildup in their arteries, which increased their odds of getting heart disease, compared with people who didn't take the supplements.

Nutritional and Other Therapies for Osteoporosis
Consider incorporating the following into your diet and daily routine:

- **Eat calcium-rich foods every day**. Good sources of calcium can be found in nondairy foods such broccoli, sesame seeds, black-eyed peas, blackstrap molasses, kale, okra, bok choy, oranges, sardines, mushrooms, poppy seeds, almonds, and figs.
- **Eat magnesium-rich foods every day**. Our menu plan is rich in these foods that include almonds, broccoli, and lentils. Pumpkin seeds and sunflower seeds are also good sources of magnesium.
- **Eat vitamin K–rich foods every day**. The best sources are leafy green vegetables (see the calcium-rich greens listed above), but most vegetables are good sources.

As much as we try, many of us don't get enough of these vitamins and minerals in our diet. If this is the case for you, I recommend the following nutrients, botanicals, and other compounds, which I prescribe to my patients diagnosed with osteoporosis, as well as for those who want to prevent the disease.

- **Magnesium supplement**. To ensure maximum absorption, take with meals and limit to 250 mg per dosage. Magnesium is also an important mineral in the bone matrix and is usually provided with calcium to offset some of its constipating effects.
- **Vitamin D**. I can't emphasize enough how much of a pivotal role vitamin D plays in facilitating the absorption of calcium, thereby helping support healthy and

strong bones. It also is an important nutrient for promoting bone mineralization, along with a number of other vitamins, minerals, and hormones (1,000 to 2,000 units a day).

- **Vitamin K.** Vitamin K helps activate certain proteins that are involved in the structuring of bone mass. Talk with your doctor about the effects of vitamin K if you are taking a blood-thinning medication.

Chronic Fatigue Syndrome

According the Centers for Disease Control and Prevention (CDC), CFS is defined by persistent fatigue that is not the result of ongoing exertion, is not alleviated by rest, and prevents people from engaging in everyday activities. CFS also has many of the same characteristics as fibromyalgia, including unexplained fatigue, poor sleep, muscle pain, poor memory, and headaches. Because there are no specific tests to confirm the diagnosis, many doctors believe, like fibromyalgia, that it is a psychological condition rather than a physical illness. At times, it is difficult to clinically distinguish the two disorders. Despite this, it is estimated that more than one million Americans have CFS, which strikes more people in the United States than multiple sclerosis and lupus.[5]

Symptoms of CFS

If you have four or more of the following symptoms that persist or recur during six or more consecutive months, you might have CFS:

- feelings of malaise lasting more than a day after physical exertion
- headaches or a new pattern or severity

- impairment in short-term memory or concentration
- multijoint pain without redness or swelling
- muscle pain
- sore throat
- tender cervical or axillary nodes
- unrefreshing sleep

Causes of CFS

Like fibromyalgia, the cause of CFS is unknown. There are many theories, however, as to why the illness develops, including

- allergies (food and environmental)
- hormonal disturbances
- infections (viral, bacterial, fungal and parasitic)
- nutritional deficiencies
- toxicity

Treatments for CFS

My experience has shown that it is not effective to use a single treatment modality to treat CFS, as one condition can trigger another (e.g., a viral illness can trigger a hormonal imbalance). A single treatment modality will not achieve the optimum results. Conventional medicine's reliance on one drug to treat an illness is not effective for this condition. Because patients with CFS have multiple problems occurring simultaneously, only a holistic approach will be effective, including antibiotic therapy, natural hormonal therapies, nutritional therapies, and detoxification.

Robert's Story

A thirty-eight-year-old pharmaceutical sales rep got a flu-like illness from which he never recovered. He was the father of two and a competitive body builder and weight lifter. He rarely got sick. After his bout with the flu, however, he couldn't get out of bed. No matter how much he tried to fight it, his fatigue got the better of him. He stopped going to work and to the gym, and he was unable to help take care of his kids. It got so bad that he was debating going on disability. He went to his doctor, who gave him a bunch of tests and told him he would get better soon. But months later, he was not better, and he still couldn't get out of bed. His doctor concluded that he must be depressed and put him on antidepressants. "I'm not depressed," he told his doctor. "I'm sick!"

Aside from the fatigue, Robert had a burning sensation in his stomach, caused by reflux in his esophagus, and alternating periods of diarrhea and constipation. He went to a gastroenterologist, who diagnosed him with IBS. When Robert asked if he should change his diet, he was told it made no difference what he ate. Instead, he was given medication to calm down his bowels, which didn't help.

When he came to see me, he was miserable. No matter how many hours he slept at night, he'd wake up tired, a classic symptom of CFS. I did my usual work-up with him, checking for vitamin, mineral, and hormone levels and performing a comprehensive digestive analysis. The results showed an imbalance of good and bad bacteria and an overgrowth of pathogenic (bad) bacteria. Unlike many of my patients, Robert's diet was good, so the trigger for him was the flu episode. I gave him a probiotic to supply him with good flora and herbal therapies combined with an antibiotic to treat the pathogenic bacteria. He also had a severe B12 deficiency, so I had him take B12 shots once or twice a week along with a multivitamin.

Within six weeks, he was able to work out lightly, and his gut was feeling much better. He gradually returned to his normal life, including going back to work, interacting with his family, and lifting weights regularly.

University Study Links Gut Bacteria to
Chronic Fatigue Syndrome
Scientists have identified a bacterial blueprint for CFS, offering evidence that it is a physical disease with biological causes and not a psychological condition, according to a 2016 article in *The New York Times*. In a study published in *Microbiome*, researchers recruited forty-eight people with CFS and thirty-nine healthy controls. Next they analyzed the quantity and variety of bacteria species in their stools and searched for markers of inflammation in their blood. The stool samples of those with CFS had significantly lower diversity of species compared with the healthy people, a finding typical of inflammatory bowel disease (IBS).

The study also revealed that people with CFS had higher blood levels of lipopolysaccharides, inflammatory molecules that might indicate that bacteria have moved from the gut into the bloodstream (classic signs of leaky gut), where they can produce various symptoms of disease. Using these criteria, the researchers were able to accurately identify more than 83 percent of CFS cases based on the diversity of their gut bacteria and lipopolysaccharides in their blood.

Finding a biomarker for CFS has been a longtime goal for researchers who hope to one day develop a diagnostic test for the condition. The importance of the study finding, says lead author Maureen R. Hanson of Cornell University, is that it might offer new clues as to why people have these symptoms.[6]

Sick and Tired? Try These Energy-Boosting Lifestyle Tips
Sick and tired of your arthritis, osteoporosis, fibromyalgia, or CFS? Instead of giving in to your exhaustion by creasing the

couch or pulling the blankets over your head, fight the fatigue by doing the following activities that are fun, stress relieving, and energy boosting:

- **The healing power of music**. Researchers have found that listening to music boosts energy and stimulates positive thinking. It also lowers our blood pressure, activates our brain's reward centers, and reduces the activity in the part of the brain associated with negative emotions. In other words, music reduces our stress. Listen to your favorite playlist on the way to work or sing along with kids or grandkids. Even more rewarding than passive listening is learning how to play an instrument or even joining band or orchestra (even if the only place you play is in your garage).

- **Straighten up**. Slouching can sap your energy (not to mention make you look as bad as you might feel). According to the International Chiropractors Association, slouching requires your muscles to work harder to hold up your body, which can lead to fatigue. Just fifteen minutes of reading or typing in a slumped-over position strains the neck, shoulders, and upper-back muscles. Incessant texting causes a newfound condition known as "tech neck." If you feel yourself slouching, imagine a string attached to the top of your head is pulling you upward and make sure that your shoulders and hips are aligned. Doing push-ups against the wall (as many as you feel comfortable doing without pain) is a safe and easy way to strengthen your back muscles.

- **Get up!** Another casualty of working long hours at a desk or chronic fatigue is sitting too long without a break. Every thirty minutes, go for a quick walk around your home or office, get a glass of water, or do a few slow stretches to get your blood circulating. Set phone alerts so you remember to get up. When you're at your desk, sit in a chair that provides good lower-back support and keep your knees slightly higher than your hips.

- **Meditate—don't medicate**. In a world rife with quick fixes and magic pills, it's nice to know there is a scientifically proven practice that can change the way you feel in as little as twenty minutes a day. Yogis and researchers agree: meditating—even just a few minutes of deep breathing—reduces anxiety and decreases depression. Setting aside time to do mini-meditations throughout the day can help when you're overwhelmed. Find a quiet spot with no distractions, sit in a relaxed position with your eyes closed, and take deep, slow breaths (in for four counts and out for four counts). Acknowledge the thoughts that enter your consciousness before letting them float away like balloons rising into the clouds while you refocus on your breathing.

- **Pep up with peppermint**. The scent of peppermint decreases fatigue by up to 25 percent, according to researchers at Wheeling Jesuit University in West Virginia. Keep a bowl of peppermints on your desk to get you through the late-afternoon slump or light a peppermint-scented candle and enjoy the energizing aroma.

- **Eat protein and veggies**. Fried and sugary foods provide a quick burst of energy but can leave you feeling hungry and depleted just thirty minutes later. Instead, eat fruits, veggies, whole grains and proteins (like nuts, if not allergic) for snacks. They help keep your blood sugar even, enabling you to avoid extreme energy highs and lows.

- **Laughter is truly the best medicine**. You've probably heard the adage that it takes more muscles to frown than to smile, which is factually correct. Also true is that laughter reduces stress, lowers blood pressure, elevates mood, and might boost the immune system. In a university study, humor associated with mirthful laughter (HAML) was shown to help alleviate symptoms from a variety of chronic medical conditions. So the next time you need a burst of energy, try watching a funny movie, video, or TV show; go to a comedy club; or connect with others who share a great sense of humor.

- **Find your sweet spot**. Acupressure techniques can be natural energy boosters, according to researchers at the University of Michigan in Ann Arbor. This technique stimulates specific points along the body using thin needles or the application of heat, pressure, or laser light. An ancient Chinese practice, acupuncture is used to treat a range of conditions, including joint pain, headaches, and digestive problems. Research also shows that the acupressure point in the center of the top of your head can have a huge impact on pumping up energy. To find the point, place your thumbs on the tops of your ears and stretch your hands up until your middle fingertips meet at the top of your head. Tap on this spot lightly while taking deep breaths.

- **Break a sweat**. The National Institutes of Health (and just about every study that has been done) says that exercise is an excellent way to rev up your energy. Work up to thirty minutes a day, if you are not used to moving. Too busy to get your heart pumping? Research has found that just ten minutes of exercise can improve mood, increase energy, and reduce feelings of fatigue. The next time you're feeling draggy, walk around the block or mall, go for a short bike ride, or swim a few laps in the pool.

- **Get hydrated**. Dehydration is a major cause of fatigue, so get out your water bottle. Water makes up about 80 percent of the brain and is an essential element in neurologic transmissions. Drinking water (half your bodyweight in ounces) won't just help your leaky gut; it'll keep you from feeling sluggish.[7]

Next I will explain the connection between gut health and the increasing rates of autoimmune diseases.

Autoimmune Diseases

As with many life-altering events, an autoimmune illness is almost guaranteed to cause you to re-evaluate your priorities.

—Joan Friedlander, author of *Women, Work, and Autoimmune Disease*

Autoimmune conditions affect more than fifty million Americans, a large percentage of whom are women. They are considered one of the leading causes of death in women under the age of sixty-five. A wide variety of illnesses are classified as autoimmune disorders, including type 1 diabetes, lupus, multiple sclerosis, Crohn's ulcerative colitis, and Hashimoto's disease, and each have different symptoms that can range from mild to severe. What is an autoimmune disorder, what causes them, and how can they be treated? And why are autoimmune diseases so prevalent in a developed country like ours with access to nutrition, modern sanitation, and advanced medical care?

You might suspect by now that the answers are somewhere in the gut—and you'd be right. I will explain the connection between dysbiosis, or an imbalanced gut flora, and the increasing rates of autoimmune diseases; the treatments and therapies that have worked for my patients; and ways that you might be able prevent or delay the onset of some of these illnesses if you are at risk.

What Are Autoimmune Diseases?

Although there are many types of autoimmune diseases that can affect different organs, what they all have in common is the immune response caused by systemic inflammation that leads your body to attack itself. Your immune system has a sophisticated method for keeping you safe. This includes identifying foreign substances that enter your body or that you come into contact with. When your immune system detects danger, it produces substances called antibodies to bind to and inactivate the harmful intruders. Autoimmune diseases are created when your body inappropriately produces antibodies against its own tissues. This can occur when the body is attempting to defend itself against something potentially harmful, such as an allergen, a toxin, or an infection. Autoimmunity can occur when the gut is inflamed, causing proteins to be absorbed into the bloodstream. These abnormal proteins can stimulate the immune system to not only produce antibodies against the food protein itself but inadvertently attack the body's own tissues. When certain types of tissues are mistaken for damaging substances, your body will turn these antibodies against itself, wreaking havoc on your organs. In other words, your body is literally attacking and destroying its own tissue.

What Causes Autoimmune Diseases?

There are many underlying factors that can cause an autoimmune condition, including an underlying genetic component. Certain genes that control the production of antibodies can be turned on by many factors, including toxins from heavy metals like mercury or mycotoxins from molds, infections like candida, the herpes simplex virus, and most significantly, chronic inflammation linked to food sensitivities—particularly gluten intolerance. There is a significant link between autoimmune diseases and gluten intolerance (thus the gut connection).

Ten Signs You Might Have an Autoimmune Disease

If you are experiencing any of the following symptoms, especially more than one or two of them, you might have an autoimmune disease:

1. abdominal pain and bloating, blood or mucus in your stool, diarrhea, or mouth ulcers
2. difficulty concentrating or focusing
3. dry eyes, mouth, or skin
4. feeling tired or fatigued, weight gain, or cold intolerance
5. hair loss or white patches on your skin or inside your mouth
6. joint pain, muscle pain, weakness, or a tremor
7. multiple miscarriages or blood clots
8. numbness or tingling in the hands or feet
9. recurrent rashes or hives, sun-sensitivity, a butterfly shaped rash across your nose and cheeks
10. weight loss, insomnia, heat intolerance, or rapid heartbeat

What Should You Do If You Suspect You Have an Autoimmune Disease?

If you suspect that you have an autoimmune disease, the most important steps to stopping and reversing your disease and symptoms are to identify and then treat the underlying cause. Conventional doctors only treat the symptoms of autoimmune diseases; often they prescribe medications such as anti-inflammatory drugs, steroids, or immunosuppressants, which fail to address the underlying cause of the condition. An autoimmune disease is not caused from a lack of anti-inflammatory drugs, steroids, or immunosuppressants. And while they might be effective in the short term, they are not a long-term solution. Treatments involving immunosuppressant drugs increase the risk of severe infections and cancer when taken for long periods of time.

Identifying which autoimmune disease you might have can be a difficult process. Symptoms can be vague because autoimmune diseases can present themselves in so many different ways, affecting the thyroid, the brain, the skin, or other organs. I suggest that you work closely with your holistic doctor when determining what is making you sick and deciding on the best treatment for you.

Treating and Reversing Autoimmune Diseases

A diagnosis of an autoimmune disease can be frightening and confusing. It doesn't help that conventional medicine only offers treatment of the symptoms, not a real solution to the disease. Pharmacologic options targeted only at inflammation in the body will not provide a long-term benefit or cure for autoimmune diseases. This is why treatments like nonsteroidal anti-inflammatory drugs (NSAIDs) and other drug therapies are doomed to fail. Additionally, the continued use of these medications is associated with a host of serious adverse side effects, such as life-threatening infections. I believe there is a gut imbalance that can lead to a bacterial infection for many autoimmune disorders, and unless the underlying cause (i.e., the infectious process) is properly treated, the illness will not improve.

One of the methods I use for my patients is to immediately place them on a comprehensive elimination diet to remove the top inflammation-causing foods. I also recommend that they remove all grains, sugars, and refined foods from their diet. As I mentioned, gluten in grains have been implicated in autoimmune diseases, as have lectins, a type of protein found in many plant foods that can cause damage to the lining of your gastrointestinal tract and interfere with metabolism when consumed in large amounts.

In order to assess my patients' gut function, I order a comprehensive stool test to look at levels of good bacteria, bad bacteria, yeast, and parasites. This test can also help diagnose leaky gut syndrome (LGS). I then apply the four *R*s (remove, replace, reinocculate, and repair; see Chapter 2) approach to healing the gut. More than 80 percent of our immune system is in our gut, so if you have an autoimmune disease, it is likely that you also have a leaky gut that needs to be repaired. Without fixing your leaky gut, you won't be able to reverse your condition.

I also check the patient's blood levels for various antibodies and look for hidden or underlying infections. After that, if the symptoms have not completely resolved, I search for toxins such as mercury and mycotoxins (chemicals produced by fungi that readily colonize crops). The World Health Organization states that there is no minimum level of mercury that does not cause harm. It binds tightly to fatty tissue of the body and to cells with sulfur groups (present in coenzymes and certain proteins). Mercury is not the only toxic-heavy metal that can negatively impact the immune system; lead, cadmium, and nickel are other metals that can cause immune system problems such as autoimmune disorders.

If I find heavy metals, I will often place the patient on oral chelation (pronounced "key-LAY-shun") treatment, which is used in conventional medicine for removing heavy metal, including mercury, from the blood. It involves intravenous injections and oral dosing of a chelating agent called ethylenediaminetetraacetic acid (EDTA). Mercury exposure can also lead to nutrient deficiencies like selenium deficiency. Selenium can be used in the body as it binds to mercury in order to remove it. It is vitally important that adequate selenium levels be maintained for any detoxification program to succeed. When dosing with selenium, 100–200 μg (micrograms) works for most patients.[1]

Diabetes

I've been helping patients with diabetes for more than thirty years, including my dad (yes, he had just about every condition in this book). It's a terrible illness, and anyone who watches a loved one go through the downward spiral of diabetes understands this. Diabetes is a group of illnesses where the pancreas does not produce enough insulin or the insulin that is being produced is not being utilized properly, resulting in high blood sugar levels over a prolonged period. The most common forms are type 1 and type 2 diabetes. Both types of diabetes increase glucose levels and, if left untreated, can cause serious complications. Diabetes currently affects more than 371 million people worldwide and is expected to affect 552 million by 2030. A new case of diabetes is diagnosed every thirty seconds in the United States.

Type 1 diabetes (T1D) tends to affect people from infancy to their thirties, typically developing when the body's own immune system attacks the pancreas and prevents the gland from producing insulin (which makes this an autoimmune condition). As many as 1.25 million Americans may have T1D, according to the American Diabetes Association.

Type 2 diabetes (T2D) typically develops after age forty but has recently begun to appear with more frequently in children due to the standard American diet causing childhood obesity. Type 2 diabetes is responsible for 90 to 95 percent of all the diagnoses of the disease. If a person is diagnosed with type 2 diabetes, their pancreas still produces insulin, but the body does not produce enough or is not able to use it effectively.

Causes of Diabetes

Scientists are still not clear about what causes diabetes, but it is clear that our diabetes epidemic is not being caused by bad genetics; it is a result of eating too much of the wrong types of foods combined with a lack of exercise. In other words, genes don't tell the whole story; environmental factors might also play a role. Type 2 diabetes is associated with obesity, older age, family history of the disease, and physical inactivity.

Table 1: Symptoms of Type 1 Diabetes

Learn to recognize the warning signs for T1D, which can save your life or someone you love. Type 1 diabetes can go undiagnosed in its early stages because the symptoms are sometimes mistaken for more common illnesses like the flu. Take notice if you or someone you know experiences the following:

drowsiness and lethargy

extreme thirst

frequent urination

(continued)

Table 1: Symptoms of Type 1 Diabetes (*continued***)**

fruity, sweet, or wine-like odor on breath

heavy, labored breathing

increased appetite

sudden vision changes

sudden weight loss

sugar in urine

stupor or unconsciousness

Call your doctor immediately if you have one or more of these symptoms.[2]

Treatments for Type 1 Diabetes

Those diagnosed with type 1 diabetes must inject insulin several times every day or continually infuse insulin through a pump. They must also clean up their diet by avoiding dairy, sugar, refined foods, and exercise or move regularly, which will help keep their weight in check and allow the insulin receptors to function optimally.

New Study Examines T1D Link to Leaky Gut

Signals from the digestive system can affect our metabolism, raising or reducing risk for health conditions like diabetes. This involves interactions between nerve signals, gut hormones and the bacteria that live in the digestive system. This theory was tested in a new study conducted at the Diabetes Research Institute in Milan, Italy.

Participants with Type 1 diabetes were shown to have inflammation of the gut and microbiome that differs from what is seen in those who do not have diabetes or even in those with other autoimmune conditions, such as celiac disease. "Some researchers have theorized that the gut may contribute to the development of type 1 diabetes, so it is important to understand how the disease affects the digestive system and microbiome," said the study's lead author, Lorenzo Piemonti, MD.

The San Raffaele Hospital study examined the microbiomes of fifty-four individuals who underwent endoscopies and biopsies of the first part of the small intestine between 2009 and 2015. Some of the volunteers were already having a procedure to diagnose a gastrointestinal disorder. "This approach allowed researchers to directly assess the gastrointestinal tract and bacteria, unlike studies that rely on stool samples for analysis," explained Dr. Piemonti. "The analysis of tissues sampled from the endoscopy produced high-resolution snapshots of the innermost layer of the gastrointestinal tract. We don't know if Type 1 diabetes' signature effect on the gut is caused by or the result of the body's own attacks on the pancreas. By exploring this, we may be able to find new ways to treat the disease by targeting the unique gastrointestinal characteristics of individuals with Type 1 diabetes."

The results of this study have yet to be published but will be keenly awaited by doctors who understand the link between LGS and autoimmune diseases.[3]

Treatments for Type 2 Diabetes

While both types of diabetes can be improved by dietary changes and exercise, type 2 diabetes can actually be reversed with nothing more than a few basic lifestyle changes. The most commonly prescribed drugs for T2D, oral medications, do little to reverse the course of this illness. In fact, most of these drugs are associated with serious adverse effects. For the majority of those with type 2 diabetes, the most effective treatments include eating a healthy diet, losing weight, correcting nutrient deficiencies, exercising, and detoxifying. Following these steps can cure type 2 diabetes in many patients. I'll take these one by one.

Food

I have no doubt that the diabetes epidemic we are currently seeing is due, in large part, to the large-scale consumption of refined foods. The glycemic index is a classification of carbohydrates based on how quickly the food is metabolized into glucose. Eating foods with a low glycemic index is beneficial for everyone and helps prevent diabetes. Examples of low glycemic foods include apples, grapefruit, and green vegetables. The glycemic index can be a good guide to use when determining the wisest food choice. I will talk more about this in Chapter 7.

Eating unrefined, healthy food products can have an anti-inflammatory effect in the gut. These include fruits, vegetables, nuts, beans, seeds, fish (wild), and eggs (from organic sources). They contain naturally occurring vitamins, minerals, proteins, fats, and enzymes that provide the body with the basic raw materials it needs to support overall health.

Exercise

If you are inclined to stay reclined, follow the plan that I've already outlined in previous chapters for introducing exercise into your life. Start moving gradually for a few minutes a day and work your way up to thirty minutes or more. It is imperative that type 2 diabetics lose weight in order to get better! Exercise can consist of simple movement like walking, which doesn't have to be done at a gym.

Hormones

I've treated many diabetic patients with natural, bioidentical hormones with excellent results, including improving their ability to lose weight and optimize blood sugar once the hormonal system is balanced. My clinical experience has shown a direct correlation between hormone irregularity and diabetes. In nearly all diabetics, adrenal and thyroid hormones are imbalanced. The adrenal glands are responsible for producing hormones that help regulate blood sugar. Dehydroepiandrosterone (DHEA), a hormone that comes from the adrenal gland, for example, has been shown to be effective in weight-loss management by increasing the oxidation of fatty acids. Studies have shown that women taking DHEA had a 10 percent decline in overall abdominal fat compared to those taking a placebo. Men experienced a 7.4 percent decline in abdominal fat compared to a placebo.

Supplements

Years of diagnosing and treating diabetics have convinced me of the importance of properly balancing supplements in diabetic patients. Diabetics are notoriously deficient in many important nutrients that provide the body with the raw materials necessary for optimizing blood sugar. In fact, I have yet to see a new diabetic patient not have multiple nutrient deficiencies.

Two of the common nutrient deficiencies in type 2 diabetics are magnesium and iodine. Studies have revealed that patients who are deficient in magnesium have a much harder time controlling their blood sugar. Some researchers speculate that a magnesium deficiency can interrupt the production of insulin and its secretion from the pancreas. Magnesium can be found in many food sources, including nuts, cocoa, tea, and leafy green veggies. I suggest asking your doctor to get your red blood cell magnesium levels checked before taking supplements. Typical doses of magnesium range from 100 to 400 mg a day.

Iodine deficiency is also occurring at epidemic rates. Iodine helps regulate the thyroid gland, and it is impossible to have a properly functioning thyroid without it. Tests have shown that iodine and thyroid hormone levels decreased in rats that developed diabetes. I have found that type 2 diabetic patients can often stop their oral medications after iodine supplementation, as their blood sugar dramatically improves. I have also been able to lower insulin doses in nearly every patient I've treated with iodine. More information about iodine can be found in my book, *Iodine: Why You Need It, Why You Can't Live without It.*

Other Nutrients

There are many other nutrients that are important for supplying diabetic patients with the necessary raw materials to help them recover from their illness. These include chromium (when taken in certain doses, chromium enables your natural insulin stores to better control your blood sugar), zinc, lipoic acid, vanadium, folic acid, cinnamon bark, and vitamins B1, B2, B3, B5, and B6. I've helped formulate a supplement called Glucoreduce, which I have found effective for diabetic patients. You can order this at http://www.medixselect.com or by calling 800-500-HEALTH.[4]

Kevin's Story

Kevin, a sixty-five-year-old retired autoworker, came to me with diabetes, which was first diagnosed fifteen years earlier. He was fifty pounds overweight and having trouble walking up stairs and doing daily activities. He was taking multiple medications for hypertension and diabetes. He had tried various diets, and he was on numerous medications to control his blood sugar, but he kept getting sicker. He told me he felt like he was going to die.

Not surprisingly, he had many gut complaints. He was constantly hungry and had bloating and stomach pains after eating. His standard American diet consisted of high-carb, high-fat, refined foods. When I talked to him about his diet, he didn't know what he should be eating and what foods he should be avoiding. I did a stool digestive analysis that showed he had dysbiotic gut flora—an abnormal amount of bad bacteria and yeast and not enough good bacteria—caused by a leaky gut.

I spent a long time talking to him about changing his lifestyle habits, including drinking water; avoiding all refined sugar, salt, and carbohydrates; and adhering to a strict diet of high-protein, high-fat, and whole foods. I put him on pre- and probiotics to feed his good bacteria. I also told to work up to walking thirty minutes a day. He didn't want to do it at first because he felt so bad and he could hardly move, but after a while, he started to enjoy the walks that became a part of his daily routine. In fact, if he had to skip a day, he felt out of sorts.

Over the next year, he gradually lost seventy-five pounds—a remarkable accomplishment. "Doc, I feel like a new man. Without making the changes you asked me to do, I would have died. I know it. I feel twenty or thirty years younger," he stated. He was able to come off all his hypertension and other medications, and most importantly, he was diabetes-free! He told me that he looked and felt like a new man. His gut was better (and smaller!), and he no longer felt bad after eating. Kevin is a classic success story of someone who changed his lifestyle by cleaning up his act (and his gut) and by getting off the couch, which cured his disease.

Lupus

Lupus is a chronic autoimmune disease that can damage any part of the body, including the skin, joints, and internal organs. When the immune system goes haywire, it's difficult to fight off viruses, bacteria, and germs that cause inflammation. Lupus is also a disease of flares, which means fluctuating symptoms come and go (sometimes you will feel ill and sometimes, in the remission stage, you will feel fine). The Lupus Foundation estimates that at least 1.5 million Americans have the disease, although the actual number might be higher because there have been no large-scale studies to show how many people in the United States are living with lupus. It can range from mild to life-threatening and should always be treated by a doctor. With good medical care, most people with lupus can lead a full life.

Symptoms of Lupus
Because lupus can affect so many different parts of the body, there are a wide range of symptoms. Certain symptoms can appear at different times, depending on the course and severity of the disease.

Treatments for Lupus
Conventional treatments for lupus include immunosuppressant drugs that are also used in chemotherapy. In addition to medications, there are alternative therapies that can be used, including homeopathy, chiropractic, traditional Chinese

Table 2: The Most Common Symptoms of Lupus

abnormal blood clotting

anemia (low numbers of red blood cells or hemoglobin, or low total blood volume)

butterfly shaped rash across cheeks and nose

extreme fatigue (tiredness)

fever

fingers turning white and/or blue when cold (Raynaud's phenomenon)

hair loss

headaches

mouth or nose ulcers

pain in chest on deep breathing

painful or swollen joints

sun- or light-sensitivity (photosensitivity)

swelling (edema) in feet, legs, hands, and/or around eyes

medicine (such as acupuncture and Tai Chi), Ayurveda, naturopathy, massage therapy, meditation, biofeedback, and herbs and other supplements. At the moment, there is not one herbal product known to significantly reduce lupus symptoms, although few studies have been done in this area. There is some evidence, however, that acupuncture can provide relief from joint pain and that

Note: Many of these symptoms occur in other illnesses. In fact, lupus is sometimes called "the great imitator" because its symptoms are similar to those of rheumatoid arthritis, blood disorders, fibromyalgia, diabetes, thyroid problems, Lyme disease, and bone diseases, among others.

meditation and biofeedback techniques can offer some relief from stress and help with pain management.

I recommend that all lupus patients have their vitamin D levels checked with a blood test. If your level is quite low, I might recommend starting with a high dose at first and then lowering the dose later. Anyone who has not had their vitamin D level checked should not use more than 2,000 international units per day, as vitamin D is fat-soluble and can build up in the body if used to excess.

LGS is part of lupus. I have found gut flora disrupted in every lupus patient that I have tested. As with all LGS-related diseases, you should always clean up your gut by eliminating sugar and processed foods and eat a whole-food diet with lots of fresh fruits and vegetables. Fresh fruits and vegetables contain many antioxidants, which help deactivate and remove toxins from the body. High-fiber foods help remove toxins from the gut. Additionally, ingredients such as cinnamon, ginger, spices found in many Indian dishes, fresh green herbs, and water all help cleanse the body. Eating a healthy diet could lessen the effects of steroids, if you are taking them, on the insulin system, although steroids often make you hungry for unhealthy foods! Do the best you can to fight the urge to eat junk food.[5]

Beating Lupus: One Woman's Story

Here's an inspirational story that a woman shared on Further food.com—an informative blog devoted to healthful eating and living—about her triumph over lupus using the food elimination method. There's nothing like being proactive with your disease!

In 2009, when I was first diagnosed with lupus, I was so upset that I fell into a state of depression. There were days when I could barely make it out of bed due to the pain and extreme fatigue. While I was prescribed medications, I still suffered from joint pain and just learned to live with it. In May 2014, I suffered a second lupus flare-up. Symptoms included extreme fatigue, fever, inflammation, and more swelling. I was initially very disappointed and upset, but this time I decided things would be different. I decided I would be in control of the disease, not the other way around. I knew I didn't want to be on multiple medications, so I decided to research how food could help my body heal. I started by researching what foods could aggravate my symptoms and began by eliminating them from my diet. Now, six months later, I'm off medications!

Lesson Learned

1. Eliminating meats and dairy products reduced my joint stiffness.
2. Eating more raw foods increased my energy.
3. Eliminating sugars and processed foods got rid of my migraines.

How I Did It

After eliminating all dairy products, meats, and refined carbs and increasing my fruit and vegetable intake, I quickly noticed how much better I was feeling. Next, I eliminated sugars, natural or man-made, and then decided to eliminate processed foods. I opted for a whole-foods diet. I ate based on foods that have been shown to boost your immune system, reduce inflammation, and improve joint health. I did learn that some foods could be healthy in one way but detrimental to me in another. I evaluated any new foods by paying close attention to how my body reacts. One thing is for sure: my dietary changes not only helped keep my symptoms at bay, but have also improved my outlook on life!

What Is There to Lose?

Yes, it takes commitment and determination to embark on such a journey, but what is there to lose? I wanted to prove to myself that I could overcome this. I wanted to prove to myself that I have lupus, but lupus does not have me. So far, the disease does not define me, and it is not what drives me anymore; instead, I am driven by the desire to live as my healthiest, optimal self, every day.[6]

Crohn's Disease and Ulcerative Colitis

Research has shown that a disrupted microbiome might contribute to the development of inflammatory bowel diseases (IBDs) such as Crohn's disease or ulcerative colitis. Scientists have also confirmed that people with IBD have a different gut microbiota composition than healthy people.

This is why these two conditions respond well to cleaning up the diet and gut. The inflammation of the colon in both cases is caused by eating nutritionally poor foods or foods one is allergic to that leave bacteria in an imbalanced state, which breaks down the stomach lining. By simply avoiding the foods that are bad for you—in particular, dairy—you will see improvement. It will take six to eight weeks for changes to occur, and if you fall off the wagon, your symptoms will return.

Conventional treatments such as chemotherapeutic drugs that reduce inflammation also weaken the immune system. One of the reasons the immune system becomes hyperfunctioning is due to leaky gut. When we eat foods that are bad for us, the gut becomes inflamed, which produces antibodies that break down the gut wall, making it leaky. The bad food simply adds fuel to the fire. The first step, of course, is to stop eating the bad food. Typical medications are potent immune-blocking drugs that can lead to life-threatening infections and even cancer.

The Crohn's/Colitis LGS Discovery

Although LGS is starting to gain traction within the medical community, the first test for it was developed in the eighties by UCLA researchers who were trying to find the cause for Crohn's disease. The researchers discovered that a leaky gut preceded inflammation, implying that the leakiness plays a key role in disease development, not just in making it worse. The principle investigator, professor Daniel Hollander, recalls, "By allowing . . . infectious or toxic substances to penetrate the intestinal barrier . . . [increased intestinal permeability could] contribute to the cascade of events that culminate in active Crohn's disease."

In another landmark study, Harvard celiac researcher Alessio Fasano, MD, found that our bodies make a protein called zonulin that essentially unzips the tight junctions that seal the intestinal lining. Although we don't know everything that stimulates the release of zonulin, we do know that certain bacteria and gluten can do it. Along with genetic factors, this creates a perfect storm to trigger autoimmune diseases such as Crohn's and colitis.

Multiple Sclerosis (MS)

Multiple sclerosis (MS) is a condition in which the lining of nerve tissues in the central nervous system gets broken down. As a result, people develop lesions on their neural pathways, causing numbness, tingling, weakness, and a host of other neurological problems. It can be a progressive disease that is extremely debilitating. Like all autoimmune disorders, MS is stimulated by an inflammatory response. In particular, this response causes the body to break down its own myelin, a mixture of proteins and phospholipids (a class of lipids that are a major component of all cell membranes) that forms a whitish, insulating sheath around many nerve fibers. This autoimmune attack on myelin leaves nerves vulnerable to degeneration.

There is a connection between myelin and gluten antibodies. MS patients inevitably do improve when they remove gluten and dairy from their diets, particularly if they are producing antibodies to any of those. In my experience, MS responds well to a holistic treatment program. This includes improving dietary habits, balancing the hormonal system with bioidentical hormones, and correcting nutrient deficiencies. I've had people go into total remission after treatment!

New Research Bolsters the Connection between Leaky Gut and MS

In a recent study published in *PLOS ONE*, researchers at Lund University in Sweden found a connection between increased permeability of the intestines and MS. This theory regarding the LGS connection to MS has been gaining popularity in the MS research community.

Shahram Lavasani, PhD, one of the study authors, told *Healthline* magazine that he has been researching this connection for the last decade. "Back then, the scientists and professionals did not believe in involvement of the gastrointestinal tract in development of 'extraintestinal' autoimmune diseases," he said. According to Lavasani, the gut was only considered important for the development of IBDs like Crohn's disease and ulcerative colitis.

Lavasani and his colleagues had already demonstrated in earlier work that probiotic bacteria can offer a certain amount of protection against MS. This led his team to study whether increased permeability of the intestines is at work in MS.

After studying the intestinal tissue from mice infected with an MS-like disease, they found not only that a leaky gut was involved but that there was also increased inflammation in the mice's intestinal mucous membranes even before they showed symptoms of MS. Researchers noticed structural changes in the membranes of the small intestines of the infected mice and an increase in inflammatory T-cells. At the same time, they noticed a drop in the number of T-cells that regulate the immune response. Those changes are commonly seen in IBD patients, but until recently hadn't been considered for anything other than gastrointestinal diseases.

Whether a dysfunctional immune system causes LGS or the other way around, addressing diet and lifestyle are beneficial because they both help regulate the immune system, restore a healthy gut, and fight autoimmune diseases.[7]

Treatments for MS

MS is typically treated with steroids, which cause myriad side effects, including ulcers, bone density loss, increased risk of infections, and heart disease. Steroids are like a hammer drug. The problem with high doses of steroids, which are helpful in acute exacerbations of MS, is that they do not appear to have a significant impact on long-term recovery. To date, other treatments have also failed to show significant improvement in long-term recovery. Unfortunately, all the MS therapies are fraught with serious adverse effects. I have seen many MS patients on these different medications, and most of them are fairly miserable with the side effects.

A relatively new drug, AMPYRA, is touted as helping MS patients with impaired balance to walk. And while I'm interested in any therapy that helps MS patients, analysis of the drug's mechanism of action and how it was studied caused me concern. AMPYRA is a broad-spectrum potassium-channel blocker. Because potassium is an intracellular element (i.e., it works within the cells), it is crucial for brain and nerve function; without adequate amounts, the nerve cells die. In fact, potassium shortage can cause a fatal illness called hypokalemia, which is characterized by cardiac abnormalities and respiratory paralysis.

As I've written in this and other books (it bears repeating), you can't block an important receptor for the long term and expect a good result. Given this fact, the long-term use of AMPYRA will likely be problematic to the patient. You might assume that the drug manufacturer had done numerous studies with AMPYRA to ensure its safety and efficacy before releasing on the market, right? Wrong. Further investigation of this drug found that "the effectiveness of AMPYRA in improving walking in patients with multiple sclerosis was evaluated in two adequate and well controlled trials involving 540 patients."

The two "adequate" trials consisted of one trial for twenty-one weeks (fourteen weeks of drug therapy) and a second trial for fourteen weeks (nine weeks of drug therapy). The FDA has now approved a potassium-channel blocker for use in MS patients based on two short studies that lasted approximately five months. MS patients will be advised by some doctors to take this drug indefinitely to help them walk better. But I say the idea of using a potassium-channel blocker is probably not a good idea for the long term. We are designed with potassium channels for a reason; we should not be using medications to block these important receptors. My best educated guess is that this drug will be associated with serious adverse effects the longer people take it. I would not advise any MS patient to try this drug until it has been thoroughly studied. Until then, its mechanism of action should cause any physician pause before prescribing it.

Instead, there are many holistic treatments for MS that I have found to be effective. First, cleaning up the diet is paramount to helping the body reverse the damage from MS. This includes avoiding artificial sweeteners. Numerous studies have pointed to a correlation between artificial sweeteners and MS. Furthermore, there are many nutrient therapies that can help MS patients achieve remission as well as improve neurologic functioning including alpha lipoic acid, vitamin C, vitamin D, L-carnitine, and B vitamins. Drinking the proper amount of water for your weight and avoiding dehydration is a must for any MS treatment plan. Finally, removing toxic elements such as mercury from the body is very helpful.[8]

Hashimoto's Disease

Hashimoto's disease is named after Dr. Hakaru Hashimoto, the twentieth-century Japanese surgeon who first recognized the disease. HD is an autoimmune disorder in which the body produces a specialized type of white blood cell (lymphocyte) that attacks the thyroid gland. This results in an inflammatory response.

The symptoms of HD are varied. A swollen gland, otherwise known as a goiter, is common. The thyroid will enlarge in size as the disease process impairs its function. The most common complaint people have is fullness in the throat area. Initially, patients might feel signs of too much thyroid hormone—hyperthyroidism. Symptoms include racing of the heart and nervousness. This is due to an inflammation of the thyroid gland, causing the gland to release much of its stored thyroid hormone. After a period of time, and after the thyroid gland essentially "burns" itself out, the hyperthyroid symptoms will give way to hypothyroid symptoms such as fatigue and coldness.

It is common for blood tests to show elevated levels of thyroid antibodies in those who suffer from HD. These antibodies include

- antithyroid antibodies
- antimicrosomal antibodies

Hashimoto's can affect people of all ages but is most common among women in their thirties and forties. Up to 2 percent of the population suffers from the disease. See Table 3 for autoimmune illnesses associated with HD.

Table 3: Autoimmune Illnesses Associated with Hashimoto's

adrenal insufficiency
chronic active hepatitis
diabetes
Grave's disease
rheumatoid arthritis
Sjögren's syndrome

Mary's Story

Mary, age thirty-six, developed thyroid problems after the birth of her second child. "After my son was born, I could not recover," she told me. "I couldn't lose weight and I couldn't get my energy level back. I kept going to the doctor and he kept telling me I was tired because I had a baby to take care of. But I knew something else was wrong."

Mary was diagnosed with Hashimoto's disease six months later. By that time, however, she had developed a goiter, and she had antibody levels in her thyroid blood tests. Mary was told her thyroid tests were normal and that she needed no treatment at that time: "My doctor told me I had to wait until the blood tests showed signs of hypothyroidism before I could begin taking thyroid medication. I told him that I already had signs of thyroid problems, including weight gain, fatigue, coldness, and other symptoms. I had also checked my basal temperature, and it was 96.6 degrees, which is a little lower than normal. But my doctor kept telling me to wait. Wait for what? I am already feeling sick."

When I saw Mary, she complained of gut pain and bloating (LGS symptoms) and had many of the clinical signs of hypothyroidism, including puffiness under the eyes; poor eyebrow growth; a thickened, coated tongue; dry skin; and slow reflexes. I put her on pre- and probiotics for her LGS and placed her on a natural, desiccated thyroid hormone (Nature-thyroid). She immediately felt better.

"It was like a cloud was lifted off of my head," she said. "I was able to think more clearly and to lose weight. Most of all, I was able to take care of my children again." Mary continued on a small dose of Nature-thyroid (45 mg per day), and she is feeling much better.[9]

Coming up, I'll discuss the links between LGS and asthma, allergies, acne, and other chronic skin conditions.

Relief for Allergies, Asthma, Acne, and Other Skin Conditions

I used to wake up at 4 a.m. and start sneezing for five hours. I tried to find out what sort of allergy I had but finally came to the conclusion that it must be an allergy to consciousness.

—James Thurber

Allergies, whether to foods, trees, grasses, weeds, molds, or dust, are an underestimated and poorly understood epidemic in this country. More than fifty million Americans suffer from allergies, according to the Asthma and Allergy Foundation. Likewise, thirty-one million Americans have been diagnosed with asthma, which is an illness associated with allergies, as are several skin conditions such as hives and rosacea (more on those later). If you are like millions who suffer from some kind of allergy and have seen multiple doctors and taken numerous medications to treat it with little or no relief, I'm going to tell you about a safe, effective, all-natural therapy that might just change your life as it did mine!

My Asthma Story

I've included many patient stories in this book, but this is *my* firsthand experience with debilitating allergies. I suffered constantly from allergies and sore throats during childhood. At age five, I developed asthma, a common respiratory condition marked by spasms in the bronchi of the lungs that make it difficult to breathe. Keep in mind, in 1968, asthma was a relatively uncommon problem. In fact, I remember being the only student in my elementary class with asthma. Now things have changed—asthma affects nearly 10 percent of US children and more than 8 percent of adults. It usually results from an allergic reaction or other forms of hypersensitivity. At least two times a year, my parents took me to the emergency room for rescue therapy after severe asthma attacks. I used inhalers and medications to help control the asthma and allergy symptoms.

As I grew older, my symptoms worsened. I always made sure I had a rescue inhaler with me at all times. I was constantly getting viral illnesses that would lead to worsening asthma symptoms. Although I was able to do everything I wanted to do, I was always on guard. I would try various allergy and asthma medications, but they always made me drowsy and dried me out. Ten years of allergy shots proved ineffective. Some asthma medications made me jittery and nervous. I went to many allergists, but they had little to offer other than more medications. Now, this is not to say the medications weren't helpful—they were. Anyone with asthma knows the feeling of struggling to breathe. Asthma medications were lifesaving for me, as they are for many asthmatic patients. Without them, I would not be alive. Period. But asthma medications do not treat the underlying cause of asthma.

What Causes Asthma?

I am not against using medications to treat the symptoms of asthma, but like many other drugs, they do not treat the underlying causes. What are those root causes, you might ask? Conventional medicine would lead you to believe that inflammation and constriction of the airways in the lungs are the causes. However, neither is responsible. Rather, they are the reactions of the lungs to allergens or irritants.

In other words, as the body (often in the case of asthma, the lungs) is exposed to an allergen, it creates an inflammatory response and perhaps constricted airways as a way to help fight the allergen. In this case, the inflammation and constriction of the lungs is the body's way of trying to not allow the allergen to move deeply into the lungs. Although asthma medications can be lifesaving, as I said, they often become less effective the longer they are used.

Back to my story. About twenty-five years ago, I set up a conference on acupuncture. During the lunch break, I voiced my frustration about treating patients with severe allergies and asthma. I found these patients very difficult to treat. Many of them reacted to so many different substances, I often felt like I was running in circles trying to help them.

One friend of mine, an acupuncturist at the conference, Dr. Libby Slocum, said she was having success treating these patients without any medications. In fact, she wasn't prescribing herbs, vitamins, or any other natural substances either. She was using acupressure. She told me about a course that teaches doctors how to help patients overcome allergies without using drugs or supplements.

I was intrigued because of my long personal history of allergies and asthma but also skeptical. (Remember when I first met that chiropractor before becoming a holistic specialist? I am wary by nature, which serves me well as a doctor.) Anyway, I questioned Libby in depth. I had known her for years, and I trusted her judgment. She told me about a course called Nambudripad's Allergy Elimination Technique (NAET).

I went to California, where the workshop was held, and I learned how Dr. Devi Nambudripad, the founder of NAET, became extremely ill while practicing chiropractic medicine. Like me, she suffered from severe allergies her whole life. In fact, she had multiple illnesses growing up, including eczema, arthritis, joint aches, bronchitis, insomnia, depression, sinusitis, migraines, and fatigue.

As she got older, she became allergic to most substances and most foods. She began to eat less and less, as she was reacting to nearly everything she consumed. (I was not her doctor, but I would have tested her for leaky gut!) At one point, she could eat only broccoli and white rice—not exactly a well-balanced diet! Eventually she became disabled and stopped working.

During various times, she would try eating different foods, but she would react with headaches, fatigue, and other symptoms. One day, nearly four years later, Dr. Nambudripad ate a carrot, which made her extremely ill. She was so sick, she felt like she was going to pass out. She gave herself an acupuncture treatment using the pressure points that would prevent her from fainting. After the treatment, she fell asleep for a while. When she awoke, she felt "completely different"—no longer sick and tired. She looked at her hand, and she was still holding the carrot. She believed she must be onto something.

After treating herself with acupuncture for the severe allergic reaction to carrots, Dr. Nambudripad had an epiphany. She had had extreme reactions to carrots in the past. After her experience using acupuncture to alleviate this reaction, however, she began to formulate a treatment plan for herself. It allowed her to change the negative reaction that carrots caused in her body. To prove it to herself, she tried to eat carrots again and had no reaction; carrots no longer bothered her. She felt like it was a miracle!

So Dr. Nambudripad began trying the same technique with all the foods that she was allergic to, which in her case was everything. She got the same result. When she treated herself with acupuncture while holding the food, her body changed. She felt like she was curing herself of her food allergies.

The end result was NAET. Dr. Nambudripad claims she has had good results in 80 to 90 percent of patients who have seen her for allergies. She even says her technique can "cure" the body of allergies permanently. My clinical experience has validated NAET as a safe and effective method for treating food and environmental allergies. So how does it work?

How NAET Works

NAET uses muscle testing as the diagnostic method to identify which substances inhibit the energetic centers of the body. It combines different treatment modalities, including applied kinesiology (muscle testing), acupuncture (use of thin needles applied to pressure points on the body's meridians), acupressure (applying various stimulation techniques to pressure points meridians), and chiropractic (treating misalignments of the joints and spinal column through physical manipulation). First, you place the item that is being tested in the palm of the patient's hand. Then each major meridian or energy center of the body is tested using applied kinesiology.

According to the theory, when a substance that the body interprets as a negative item is placed in the patient's energy field (in this case, the hand), it can disrupt the normal flow of energy through the meridians. This disrupted energy flow is detected through a muscle test that was developed by Michigan chiropractor Dr. George Goodhart in the sixties. Since then, many chiropractors have successfully used this muscle test. It is based on the principle that the body's energetic field responds to everything in its environment. This includes pollens, temperature, people you associate with, emotions, and many other elements. These things manifest themselves in a variety of symptoms, from a runny nose and sneezing to chest pain and headaches.

By contrast, traditional medicine's view of an allergy is that it is an overreaction of the immune system to an allergen. For example, you might experience a runny nose and sneezing in the early fall as the allergen ragweed is released into the air. The conventional treatment for this problem is to use antihistamines to block histamine receptors and relieve the symptoms. While the medications will successfully treat the symptoms, it does not get to the underlying cause of the illness. Additionally, the medications can have adverse effects, such as foggy brain and drowsiness. I believe the underlying problem in the case of hay fever is an abnormal response by the body to a substance (hay fever allergen) that is harmless to a majority of people. In this case, the body is interpreting exposure to the hay fever allergen as something that is dangerous. In NAET theory, the body is misinterpreting the allergen as a dangerous substance, and the end results are the runny nose and sneezing, which is the body's way of releasing this substance and not letting it go to a deeper energetic level. By identifying the affected meridians and treating them with NAET, you can train the body not to react to the hay fever allergens (or whatever you are allergic to).

If everything is functioning optimally in your body, your energetic field will be strong. If the body senses that something might harm it, it shuts down various meridians to keep that offending item from going deeper and causing a more severe reaction or injury. This is a good thing because you don't want allergens to cause severe problems in your body. In other words, your body can respond either positively or negatively to everything in its environment. This is nature's own defense mechanism, much like antibodies defend against substances in the body that are not supposed to be there when you have a leaky gut.

There are many knockoffs of NAET and programs that claim to "speed up" the NAET protocols. I have seen these different regimens, and some are effective in their own right. But this does not take away from NAET, which has stood the test of time, having been around for twenty-five years. Dr. Nambudripad has trained tens of thousands of health care practitioners in her technique, which is still being used all over the world.

My NAET Experience

If you have a leaky gut and you are allergic to dairy, for example, you might react with a rash, diarrhea, or a headache; this is your body's way of telling you to stay away from that type of food. And if your body is continually being exposed to foods and other substances that it is allergic to, it can wreak havoc on your health.

I have seen numerous patients who have had a number of allergies. They are reacting to many things in their environment. Some of these allergic patients can eat only a few foods, like Dr. Nambudripad, because they are so sensitive to many different ones. These patients are often referred to as suffering from "multiple-chemical sensitivity," the worst kind of an allergic response. Not only have I successfully treated patients with multiple-chemical sensitivity using NAET; I was able to treat myself!

I took my introductory class on NAET in California in 1996. The first day of the course, I was talking with another doctor. We both questioned the validity of NAET. "How can you 'cure' allergies with acupressure?" we asked. I was beginning to regret the trip, and I was certain the technique was doomed to fail (remember, I am a skeptic).

The second day of the course, however, I awoke with a bad headache. I don't get headaches often, but when I do, I really suffer. I was tired and feeling a little sick to my stomach in addition to the pounding in my head. Before the class started, Dr. Nambudripad asked whether people had any physical issues. I raised my hand and told her about my headache. She asked me, "What's causing your headache?"

"It's a sinus headache. I always get it when the weather is changing," I said.

She reminded me that I was in California and that the weather rarely changes and that on that very day, it had not changed. She tested me for various substances and told me I was allergic to the salt I had on the french fries from the previous evening's meal. I thought that was interesting because I hadn't told her what I had eaten for dinner, but by using NAET, she came to the conclusion that I had salt with my meal. I had, in fact, eaten salted french fries—something I did not do often! Dr. Nambudripad gave me an acupressure treatment for the salt, and before I turned over, my headache was gone. Now she had my full attention.

A Life-Changing Treatment

I went home from that class energized by what I had learned and experienced. I immediately began treating my patients as well as myself for various allergies. In my own case, I have been allergic to dairy products since I was a child. I would wheeze and get a stuffy nose with any exposure to dairy. After one NAET treatment for dairy, I no longer had problems with it. Today I can eat dairy without having a problem, but I don't because I know that it is not good for my gut.

But it wasn't just dairy that gave me a problem. I was allergic to pollens, trees, grasses, and weeds. After years of allergy shots, NAET helped me with all the environmental allergens that once bothered me. In addition to personally experiencing the benefits of NAET, I have two practitioners who use it to treat patients in my office. I continue to recommend it to all my patients with allergies. To find a NAET practitioner in your area, go to http://www.naet.com or call Dr. Nambudripad at 714-523-8900.

The Healing Power of Acupuncture

I've discussed a little about acupuncture already, but the following is a deeper explanation about this ancient Chinese practice. Acupuncture, which has been around for five thousand years, is based on the concept of energy flow. Over time, there have been studies on its efficacy, and the American Medical Association (AMA) has accepted it as a viable treatment for a variety of conditions. The idea is that the body is made up of various energetic points (i.e., "meridians"). Each acupuncture point is like an energy center. By placing thin needles along these energy points, you can manipulate the energy flow of the body. A meridian is a specified pathway where energy, or qi (pronounced "chee"), flows. For example, there are acupuncture points that make up the liver or kidney meridians. By stimulating these acupuncture points, you can manipulate the energy of the liver and kidney meridians.

The main theory behind acupuncture is that health occurs when energy of the body is flowing normally. I describe this to my patients like the power grid that supplies electricity to our houses. When everything is working, our houses get the proper amount of electricity. When there is a storm, the power can go out in certain neighborhoods. Acupuncture theory would say that when our qi is flowing correctly, all the various organs of the body (the meridians, in acupuncture theory) are functioning normally.

When energy, or qi, is not flowing well, however, there are imbalances in the body. These imbalances are manifested as disease. When the normal energy flow of the body is restored, healing and overcoming illness can take place. This theory of energy flow is not unique to acupuncture or to Chinese medicine. Conventional medicine recognizes the concept of energy flowing through the body through electrocardiograms (ECGs), which measure the electrical activity of the heart. Electroencephalograms (EEGs) measure the electrical activity of the brain.

In addition to the AMA, the National Institutes of Health concurs that "there is sufficient evidence of acupuncture's value to expand its use into conventional medicine and to encourage further studies of its physiology and clinical values."

Hetty's Story

When I first met Hetty, she was fifty-nine years old. She told me thought she'd been poisoned while working as a dental hygienist, where she was exposed to lots of chemicals. Hetty also informed me that she was a single mother of a special needs child and that she had to get well in order to take care of her son.

On that first visit, I began to use NAET to diagnose the allergies and energy disturbances in her body. It turned out that Hetty was allergic to nearly everything. It was as if her body was totally out of sync with the world she was living in. Using drugs wasn't an option; she reported having adverse reactions to nearly all of them. Hetty was suffering from fatigue and gastrointestinal symptoms such as severe constipation, bloating, and abdominal pain. I diagnosed her with leaky gut syndrome (LGS) that was being caused, in large part, from her exposure to dental chemicals and her inflammation from food allergies.

NAET was definitely the best and safest treatment for Hetty. Next we started treating her for the chemicals she was exposed to at work. When I treated her for fluoroethane, an anesthetic commonly used in dentistry, she became extremely ill. She couldn't leave my office for two hours because she was too tired and dizzy, but she eventually recovered. During the time she was in one of my exam rooms, the room developed a deep chemical smell. I believe Hetty was detoxing the fluoroethane and other dental chemicals through her pores that had been stored up and was toxifying her body.

Hetty's case is not unique; there have been case histories reported in medical literature about toxic substances coming out of a patient's skin. I have seen many examples of this in my practice when my patients undergo detoxification. Hetty had a similar reaction when I treated her for nitrous oxide, another common chemical used by dentists.

It took three weeks for the NAET treatments to reverse the problems of the chemical allergies from which Hetty was suffering. This included her LGS as well. After Hetty recovered, I sent her for certification for NAET, and she worked in my office doing NAET on my patients for the next thirteen years. "NAET gave me my life back," Hetty says. "I would not be here if it weren't for NAET. I felt like I was dying. Now I can pay it forward by helping others to change their lives and get better!"

Gut Reactions to Food Allergies

As you now know, when you have a leaky gut, the intestinal barrier becomes compromised, allowing toxins and other pathogens to get absorbed through openings in the lining. In a healthy gut, this barrier selectively lets digested nutrients enter the small intestine when it is ready to accept them. With LGS, however, nutrients can be absorbed before they are fully digested. When this happens, the body's immune response through specific antigen-antibody markers will identify some of these foods as foreign irritants.

After a particular food touches the lining of cells that cover the exterior surfaces of the body, an inflammatory immune response is initiated, which further damages the intestinal lining. So what might have started as a candida irritation (yeast overgrowth), for example, can become active inflammation every time you eat a particular food.

Some of the most common food allergies include dairy, eggs, gluten grains (wheat, oats, rye), corn, beans (especially soy), sugar, and nuts (see Table 1). Exposure to a significant allergy can sabotage treatment designed to heal the intestinal lining. For example, one might be compliant in restricting wheat, dairy, and eggs but then compromise the treatment by having sugar. In addition to using NAET to find your food allergies, I recommend trying an elimination diet in the early stages of treatment.

Table 1: Most Common Food Allergies

The following cause about 90 percent of food allergy reactions:

eggs

fish (mostly in adults)

gluten

milk

peanuts

shellfish (mostly in adults)

soy

tree nuts (walnuts, almonds, pine nuts, Brazil nuts, and pecans)

wheat and other grains with gluten (barley, rye, and oats)[1]

Food Allergy and Depression
In my experience, there is also a relationship between food allergies and depression. Eating foods that are allergenic is stressful for the body. Food allergies can manifest in a number of ways, including a runny nose and sneezing, headaches, asthma, hives, as well as depression or chest pains.[2] I'll explain more about this mind/body connection in the next chapter.

What Is Anaphylactic Shock?

When exposed to something you are allergic to, such as peanuts or a bee sting, some people experience a reaction called anaphylaxis. When this happens, the immune system releases chemicals that flood the body, which can lead to anaphylactic shock. If your body goes into anaphylactic shock, your blood pressure will drop suddenly and your airways narrow, preventing you from breathing normally. This is a potentially life-threatening condition that requires immediate medical attention.

Symptoms of Anaphylactic Shock
The symptoms include

- abdominal pain
- a sense that something is wrong with your body
- confusion
- dizziness
- feeling like you have a lump in your throat or difficulty swallowing
- loss of consciousness
- nausea, vomiting, or diarrhea
- runny nose and sneezing
- skin reactions such as hives, flushed skin, or pale skin
- difficulty breathing
- suddenly feeling too warm
- swollen tongue or lips
- weak and rapid pulse
- tingling hands, feet, mouth, or scalp
- wheezing

If you think you or someone you know is experiencing anaphylaxis, seek medical attention immediately by calling 911.

What Are the Causes and Risk Factors of Anaphylaxis?
Anaphylaxis is caused by an overreaction of your immune system to an allergen, or something your body is allergic to. In turn, anaphylaxis can result in anaphylactic shock.

Common triggers for anaphylaxis include

- certain medications such as penicillin
- insect stings
- foods such as tree nuts, shellfish, milk, and eggs
- agents used in immunotherapy
- latex

Sometimes a cause for this reaction is never identified. This type of anaphylaxis is called idiopathic.[3]

Food Intolerances

With the exception of celiac disease, food intolerances do not involve the immune system. Although food intolerances might cause some of the same symptoms as a food allergy, they cannot trigger anaphylaxis. Common intolerances include the following:

- **Gluten sensitivity**. An adverse reaction to gluten. This chronic digestive disease requires a lifelong restriction of gluten, which is found in wheat, rye, barley, and oats. When people with celiac disease eat gluten, they experience an immune reaction in the small intestine. This immune response in celiac disease might damage the lining of the small intestine, preventing proper absorption of the nutrients in food. Celiac disease is a known cause of LGS symptoms, including bloating and gas, diarrhea, constipation, headaches, itchy skin rash, and pale mouth sores.

- **Lactose intolerance.** Lactose intolerance occurs when a person's small intestine does not produce enough of the lactose enzyme, lactase. As a result, affected individuals are not able to digest lactose, a type of sugar found in dairy products. The symptoms of lactose intolerance typically occur within thirty minutes to two hours after ingesting dairy products.

For more information about celiac disease, visit http://www .celiac.org and http://www.celiaccentral.org.

Know Your Food Triggers

To pinpoint the foods that are causing your food intolerance or food allergy symptoms, you need to do some detective work through either NAET or an elimination diet. Here's how it's done:

- First, write down everything you eat or drink in a typical week. Include how much and the time of day, how the food was prepared (if not bought already cooked), and how you feel after eating it. Do this for twenty-four to thirty-six hours.
- Second, start your elimination diet by removing common foods from your diet—one at a time—for six weeks per food item. As I said earlier, it takes that long for the body to stop producing antibodies to fight the allergens. Write down any improvement in

your symptoms and make a note of which food elimi-
nations resulted in the improvements.

- If your food allergies are severe, once you've identified what food or foods trigger(s) the reaction, remove
them completely from your diet.

- If your food allergies are mild to moderate, you can
begin reintroducing foods to retest and confirm your
food triggers and to reevaluate your body's immune
system response to them (remember Dr. Nambudripad and the carrot). To do this, add each of your
trigger foods back into your diet, one per day. Eat the
suspected trigger food as part of at least two meals
that day, but be careful not to include other potential
allergens, or the results will be flawed. Record the date
and time you reintroduced each food and note both
immediate and delayed reactions that you have.

- If you experience a reaction to a particular food,
eliminate it completely from your diet. Before you
reintroduce any new food, make sure that you have
been symptom-free for at least two days. Repeat this
testing with all your possible trigger foods until you
figure out exactly which ones are causing your food
intolerance or food allergies.

Boost Low Stomach Acid

I talked about this in the digestive chapter, but inadequate
production of hydrochloric acid by the stomach might also be
the cause of food allergy symptoms. When there isn't enough
acid in the stomach to properly break down food, "foreign"
food protein molecules can cause LGS by causing inflammation of the tight junctions of the gut mucosa, allowing these
food particles to reach the bloodstream and provoke an allergic

reaction (what happens in LGS). If this is the case for you, I recommend supplementing with hydrochloric acid pills with meals (see your doctor for the right dosing). Achlorhydria, or low stomach acid production, is a common problem in those with thyroid disorders, autoimmune illnesses, and nutrient deficiencies (vitamin B12, iodine, and salt).

Enzymes

An insufficient supply of digestive enzymes is another often ignored cause of food allergies and food intolerances because the body can't properly digest foods without them. In this case, the improperly digested food particles can cause inflammation of the gut lining, leading to LGS. To improve your ability to breakdown foods, try taking two tablets of digestive enzymes (sometimes called pancreatic enzymes) about ten minutes before meals and two more about ten to fifteen minutes following a meal. I have found taking plant enzymes with meals allows digestion to start in the stomach and helps the pancreatic enzymes do the "finishing" work. The more food is thoroughly digested, the less it will be fermented in the gut. Food fermentation causes "bad" bacteria and yeast to proliferate at the expense of "good" intestinal bacteria. Plus, the more carbohydrates are digested, the lower the potential for food-inducing bad bacteria. Another benefit of enzymes is that more nutrients can be absorbed from the food we eat.

Contraindications (Caveats) for Enzyme Supplements

Enzymes should not be used under the following circumstances: active stomach or duodenal ulcers, severe bowel inflammation (characterized by blood in stools), hemophilia and other bleeding disorders, or within a week of scheduled surgery. Those with known anaphylactic allergic reactions to fungal proteins should not ingest fungal-derived enzymes.[4]

Nutritional Support for Allergies

The following nutrients strengthen your body's ability to tolerate allergenic foods without overreacting to them:

- high-potency daily multinutrients
- bioflavonoids—500 to 1,000 mg twice a day
- mineral-buffered vitamin C—2,000 to 5,000 mg a day in divided doses (Cut back if you experience stomach upset or diarrhea.)
- pantothenic acid—250 to 500 mg twice a day
- flaxseed oil—1 to 2 tablespoons per day
- unrefined salt
- adequate hydration

The Gut/Skin Connection

Frequently, when a patient walks into my office, I can tell that there is something going on in their gut by looking at their skin. The reason for this is the gut/skin connection, which scientific research has shown to be a factor:

- Studies have found that more than half of all acne sufferers have gut flora disruptions, which affect their skin (in addition to making them bloated).
- Cultures that eat a diet with little or no processed or sugary foods have fewer digestive problems and virtually no acne!

Rosacea (see page 147) has been linked to inflammation and bacterial imbalances in the gut and is one of the most common skin conditions I see in LGS patients. The reason for this is that your skin is like your intestines—everything you eat eventually shows up on it, and an unhappy gut can produce angry skin. In addition to bloating, food allergies, and food intolerances, LGS can cause both systemic and local inflammation, which results in dark circles under the eyes, blemishes, rashes, itchy skin, eczema, rosacea, and psoriasis (see the following sections).

Acne

Acne is the most common skin disorder in the United States, affecting more than seventeen million people. It can be a debilitating, scarring, disfiguring condition that anyone at any age, gender, or ethnicity can get at any time (acne is not just for teenagers).

What Causes Acne?

Acne is a skin condition that frequently occurs on the face, chest, or back. It is caused by a combination of factors: overactive sebaceous glands increase oil production, the pores become plugged by the oil, and finally, bacteria become trapped. The plugged follicle that stays beneath the skin and continues to grow is known as a whitehead (closed comedo). A comedo that reaches the surface of the skin is called a blackhead. Picking at or popping these lesions will increase the risk of infection and scarring. Hormones and heredity play a large part in whether you get acne, and stress can exacerbate breakouts.[5]

Cara's Story

Cara, a typical sixteen-year-old, was upset with her frequent acne breakouts that made her feel self-conscious and shy. She had been on several courses of antibiotics, but when she went off, the acne would come back. I took a dietary history, and she complained of stomachaches and pains that caused her to miss a lot of school. She was diagnosed with IBS with bouts of diarrhea.

Cara was eating a standard American diet full of carbs, dairy, and gluten and not a lot of whole foods, fruits, or vegetables.

I did a stool digestive analysis and found an overgrowth of clostridia bacteria, which is a pathogen. I treated her with pre- and probiotic supplements to replenish the good bacteria and spent a lot of time counseling her on eating a healthful, whole-food diet free of all refined foods including sugars, oils, flours, and oats. I told her to eat more fruits and vegetables and to drink more water. I also treated her with oregano oil, which has a potent antibiotic effect in the gut for dysbiotic (bad) bacteria. Within two weeks of being on the diet, her acne was better. Within four weeks, she was 80 percent better, and she had minimal acne that she could live with. Her gut inflammation was gone, she had no more diarrhea, and she was also thinking clearer.

Rosacea

If you are one of those people who blush easily and turn "beet red" when you are embarrassed, or you break out after eating certain foods or drinking alcohol, then you might be one of the millions who are prone to a disorder called rosacea. This is a condition where anything that causes the blood vessels in the skin to open (dilate) can lead to diffuse redness of the face, a rash that looks just like acne, and broken blood vessels. Most forms of rosacea are more common in women than in men and can occur in any ethnicity. The majority of people with rosacea are between forty and sixty years old. It's important to have an evaluation of redness of the face because there are several possible conditions that can cause this, some of which can be serious, and early evaluation and treatment can make a big difference in outcome.

Rosacea Treatments

Your dermatologist can help you with prescription treatments, but you also need to be extra careful with the skin-care products you use at home. Generally, it's good to avoid products with fragrance because they don't add value to the skin care and they can in some cases trigger rosacea.[6]

Psoriasis

Psoriasis is a chronic skin disorder characterized by periodic flare-ups of red plaques covered by a flaky surface. The most common type is known as plaque psoriasis, thick patches that frequently appear on the elbows, knees, scalp, lower back, buttocks, and navel.

While we don't know what causes psoriasis, there seems to be a combination of factors that contribute to breakouts. It typically starts with inflammation in the skin that prompts new skin cells to develop. In normal cell growth, keratinocytes (epidermal skin cells that produce keratin that helps form hair and nails) move from the bottom layer to the skin's surface and then shed, a process that takes about a month.

If you have psoriasis, the keratinocytes multiply quickly and travel from the lower layer of the skin to the surface in just three or four days. Because the skin can't shed these cells fast enough, they build up, which leads to thick, dry patches of dead skin that form plaques. Underneath, the nerves, blood, and lymphatic vessels become red and swollen.

Psoriasis Treatments

Cleaning the gut can help, but it's difficult to eradicate psoriasis entirely, although it can get at least 50 percent better by cleaning up the diet.

Eczema

This chronic skin condition tends to run in families. Much like an allergy, it is due to sensitivity in the skin and involves scaly and itchy rashes and inflammation. Eczema is common in infants and young children, where it can go away in time, but it can be chronic in adults. Like its cousin psoriasis, eczema is aggravated when people scratch the infected area, causing the skin to become thicker and itchier.

Eczema Treatments

Treating eczema starts with stopping the scratching and possibly finding the root cause that is making you itch. Keep the area dry by using mild cleansers, avoiding washcloths, and applying rich moisturizers to damp skin as soon as you get out of the bath or shower. Topical anti-inflammatories such as cortisone creams also help, so ask your doctor about what's right for you.

Also, people with eczema, especially babies, are particularly reactive to dairy and gluten. They need to go dairy- and gluten-free to clear up LGS. Babies get the milk or gluten antigens from their mothers when breastfeeding, and it crosses over into their intestines, which inflames the gut and causes the leaking. When the body gets overwhelmed, it creates an inflammatory condition. This inflammatory state can manifest as the flaky, scaly lesions found in eczema.

Apryl's Story

Apryl started getting eczema at about two months. Her mother took her to a pediatrician, who treated her with steroid creams and washes. The baby was miserable and had to wear mittens so she didn't scratch herself at night. She had scaly, weepy lesions all over her body. Apryl was breastfed from birth. I took a dietary history from the mom, who was drinking milk and eating lots of cheese. She also had a long history of asthma. I talked to her about doing testing for a dairy allergy. She didn't want the tests, but she was interested about whether the dairy could be causing the skin condition—I told her it could. She stopped consuming dairy that day, and the eczema was 50 percent better. It was the first time Apryl showed improvement without drugs. When I saw her again several months later, the eczema was all gone.

Hives

Hives are red, itchy, raised areas of skin that appear in varying shapes and sizes and typically last between six and twelve hours. Hives can be brought on by allergies, but it is often difficult to pinpoint their exact cause. Anything can cause hives, including drugs, heat, cold, change in weather, and stress. If the underlying cause is food allergies, however, they will go away as you eliminate the offending substance from your diet. NAET and the elimination diet also work well for this condition.

Joyce's Story

Joyce is a forty-five-year-old teacher who flies up from Florida to see me about once a year. She suddenly developed a case of hives out of the blue. The red, itching bumps would come and go on various parts of her body such as her arms, back, and chest. She took over-the-counter (OTC) allergy medication, but the hives just got worse over time. She'd been to a dermatologist and an allergist, who did a skin test for food allergies and found nothing. She was put on round after round of steroids and antihistamines that made her drowsy. No one could tell her the cause, so they just treated the symptoms. By the time she saw me, she was miserable from itching. Joyce ended up using NAET and discovered that she was highly sensitive to sugar. I did three treatments, and after the third, her hives finally disappeared and never returned.

The Yeast of Your Problems (Candida)

Fungal (yeast) overgrowths—such as overgrowths of candida—occur mostly in damp places, such as under your arms, in your groin, in your mouth, and elsewhere. Problems it can cause include acne, eczema, hives, athlete's foot, ringworm, and dandruff. Yeast overgrowth in the body also causes bloating and gas because yeast species are involved in fermentation of food, a process that produce carbon dioxide gas.

Imbalances that show up on the skin and scalp can profoundly affect your appearance. If you've take lots of antibiotics or steroids, you might have a yeast overgrowth that cause folliculitis, leading to hair loss and a red, scaly scalp. Identifying the cause of your bacterial imbalance and correcting it is an essential step in improving both your bloating and any associated skin or scalp conditions. We need healthy amounts of essential bacterial in our GI tract and on our skin in order for them to function well. Avoid antibiotics unless absolutely necessary because they can wipe out the healthy colonies of good bacteria in the gut and allow yeast to overgrow. Also avoid antibacterial soap that washes away healthy bacteria on the skin, which is just as essential.

Take Care of the Skin You're In

- **Avoid a "chemical spill."** Beware of products that are full of chemicals because they can destroy the delicate ecosystem on your skin. Many of the ingredients found in expensive skincare products have strange-sounding, scientific names. This is simply marketing, much like cereals that claim to be "all natural" or "healthy" but are really highly processed junk food. As food expert and author Michael Pollan once wrote, "Don't put anything in your mouth with more than five ingredients, or ingredients you can't pronounce."[7] The same goes for your skin. Chemicals like sodium lauryl sulfate (SLS) put in shampoo and cleaning products to produce lather can be easily absorbed through your skin, which will irritate it and strip away its essential oils and moisture. SLS can get absorbed into your intestines and lead to inflammation and bloating.

- **Use edible products.** Like your gut, your skin is a porous membrane that absorbs what you put on it, which ends up inside of you. A good rule of thumb is to apply the same philosophy you would when cooking. Use high-quality, simple ingredients that come from nature, not a laboratory. Raw honey, papaya, oatmeal, and coconut oil are all great for your skin.

- **Nourish your skin.** Nourish your microbiome by creating an environment for food bacteria to flourish in your gut and on your skin. This includes avoiding unnecessary antibiotics and eating lots of high-fiber foods. Pre- and probiotics containing large amounts of healthy bacteria like lactobacillus and bifidobacterium can be eaten or taken in pill, powder, or liquid form. You will notice an improvement in your gut and on your skin within thirty days.

- **Use soap and water against germs.** The proliferation of antibacterial products, including hand sanitizers, can strip away the essential oils that moisturize your body. Rinsing with soap and water (singing "Happy Birthday" twice to yourself is the right amount of time to soap up) will keep your hands sufficiently clean and healthy. Also, showering in lukewarm water is better than hot, which will dry your skin and make your hives or rosacea worse.

- **Go for the glow**. Exercise is one of the best ways to give your skin that healthy glow that comes with increasing blood flow and the release of feel-good endorphins. Dancing, running, brisk walking, yoga, tennis, swimming, and sex (think "afterglow") are all good ways to reduce bloating through rhythmic contractions of your GI system (called peristalsis).

The Way to Healthier Skin Is through the Stomach

There are natural, nutritional ways to improve the health of your skin and keep you looking younger longer. No surprise, it's all about eating the right foods (and using a broad-spectrum sunscreen of 30 SPF or more). Here are some tips that I'll talk more about in the next chapter:

- **Go green**. Perhaps the single best food group for healthy skin is dark green vegetables. It has water galore and is high in vitamin C that helps the body produce skin-tightening collagen. I say kale Caesar—or, better yet, kale with cold-pressed extra virgin olive oil and balsamic vinegar dressing.
- **Omega-3 fatty acids and flavonoids**. Both these nutrients are good for maintaining optimal blood flow to and from your skin cells. Foods that are naturally rich in omega-3 fatty acids include dark green leafy veggies, raw walnuts, wild salmon, flaxseed, and free-range, humanely raised eggs. Foods that are naturally rich in flavonoids include lettuce, cherries, citrus, cabbage, kale, spinach, goji berries, asparagus, and raw cacao.
- **Vitamin A, carotenoids, healthy fats**. Vitamin A is one of the best micronutrients for your skin. Foods

that are rich in carotenoids and healthy fats include dark green, yellow, and orange veggies such as spinach, carrots, and sweet potatoes.

- **Avoid sugar**. Processed sugar causes dysbiosis and yeast overgrowth and promotes insulin release that is associated with inflammation in the gut and on the skin.
- **Eat unrefined salt and avoid refined salt**. Refined salt has no minerals in it and has toxic ingredients such as ferrocyanide. Unrefined salt is a better choice, as it has more than eighty minerals in it.
- **Gut the gluten**. This is not the first time you're reading this, but gluten-containing grains have been associated with bloating, rashes, and even hair loss. Even if you don't have celiac disease, gutting the gluten that's in wheat, rye, and barley can do wonders for breakouts, thinning hair, and GI distress.
- **Limit your alcohol**. Did you know that alcohol is a cousin of formaldehyde, a highly toxic substance? Much less scary is that it can cause bloating (ever heard of a beer belly?) and blotchy skin and accelerate the aging process.
- **Be dairy wary**. Again, studies have shown that there is an increase in acne breakouts in people who consume lots of dairy. It also causes bloating, especially in people who are lactose intolerant. Most people could do well to avoid dairy.
- **Water for chocolate**. Here's the good news. It's a myth that chocolate causes acne flares. Dark chocolate actually has some health benefits if eaten in moderation, and the less sweet and bitter, the better. But as I've been saying throughout this book, one of the

best things you can do for your skin is to hydrate, hydrate, and hydrate (with water). Avoid caffeine and soda that will dry out your skin.[8]

Next, are you depressed, anxious, hyperactive, or foggy brained? Learn why your gut might be at the root of these and other mental disorders.

Gut Health Equals Brain Health

I regard the brain as a computer which will stop working when its components fail.

—Stephen Hawking

Stress and depression can contribute to a variety of GI conditions, such as irritable bowel syndrome (IBS), but did you know that the reverse is also true? In this chapter, I will explain how what's going on in your gut can also affect your brain, including your mood and your memory. The gut can also be linked to Alzheimer's disease, attention deficit disorder (ADD), and even autism.

Have you ever "gone with your gut" when making a decision or felt "butterflies in your stomach" when nervous? When this happens, you're probably getting signals from your "gut brain." What do I mean by this? Hidden in the walls of the digestive system, this gut brain is the link between digestion, mood, mental health, neurological conditions, and even the way you think. The scientific name for this other brain the enteric nervous system (ENS). The ENS is composed of two thin layers of more than one hundred million nerve cells lining your entire gastrointestinal tract.

What Does the Gut Brain Control?

Unlike the big brain in your head, the ENS can't do math or help you compose an e-mail. "Its main role is controlling digestion—from swallowing to the release of enzymes that break down food to the control of blood flow that helps with nutrient absorption—to elimination," says Jay Pasricha, MD, director of the Johns Hopkins Center for Neuro-gastroenterology (the study of the brain, the gut, and their impact on GI disorders). "The enteric nervous system doesn't seem capable of thought as we know it, but it communicates back and forth with our big brain—with profound results."

According to Dr. Pasricha, the ENS might trigger emotional shifts experienced by people suffering from IBS, constipation, diarrhea, bloating, and stomach pain. These findings show that irritation in the gastrointestinal system, such as leaky gut syndrome (LGS), might send signals to the central nervous system that trigger mood changes. This evidence explains why so many people with IBS and LGS develop depression and anxiety.[1]

Another study from the University of Exeter Medical School in England and the University of Zaragoza in Spain, published in the journal *PLOS ONE*, confirmed that microorganisms living in our gut help regulate our brain chemistry. The bacteria and other microbiota that reside in our gut play a key role in regulating everything from digestion and metabolism to immune function and even mood, though the mechanisms of this action remain largely a mystery. But before I explain more about the connection between gut health and mental health, let me give you some background on how the brain works.

What Is Serotonin?

Our brains are controlled by chemicals called neurotransmitters—serotonin being one of them. Neurotransmitters are the substances produced in the brain that allow it to do all the things that the brain was designed to do, including thinking, feeling, regulating mood, and controlling sleep, hunger, satiety, and more. The brain cannot function without an adequate supply and balance of neurotransmitters (see Table 1). Serotonin is one of the "feel-good" neurotransmitters. In fact, more serotonin is produced and used in the brain than any other neurotransmitter.

Table 1: Examples of Neurotransmitters

adrenaline	histamine
dopamine	noradrenaline
gamma-aminobutyric acid (GABA)	serotonin

What is not as well known is that nearly 90 percent of the body's serotonin stores are in the intestinal tract, where it plays a critical role in the digestion process. Although all neurotransmitters help regulate different behaviors, serotonin controls appetite; alcohol, drug, and nicotine cravings; gastrointestinal effects; blood flow; impulse control and aggression; mental functioning; migraines and other headaches; mood; motivation; and the sleep/ wake cycle.

Microbes Manipulate Serotonin Levels

Studies conducted in cell cultures of living mice by the Foundation for the Study of Inflammatory Bowel Diseases found that in addition to carrying signals for the brain, serotonin also plays a role in controlling bowel function. Researchers identified the protein TLR2 as the one that helps regulate levels of serotonin. These findings suggest that certain gut microbes can, through the action of TLR2, modulate levels of serotonin, directly influencing human physiology and brain chemistry.

Does this mean that the gut microbiome can also affect serotonin levels, causing changes in our mood or brain function? Absolutely. A 2014 review of the evidence into whether gut microbes can influence human emotions and behavior, published in the journal *BioEssays*, concluded that there is strong theoretical support for this notion. For example, some microbes can release chemicals that change the activity of the vagus nerve, which runs from the gut to the brain. "Microbes have the capacity to manipulate behavior and mood by altering the neural signals in the vagus nerve, changing taste receptors, producing toxins to make us feel bad, and releasing chemical rewards to make us feel good," explained the study's senior author, Athena Aktipis.[2]

Depression

Depression is a serious health problem, with symptoms that include sadness, dramatic weight gain or loss, insomnia, loss of energy, and suicidal thoughts (see Table 2). According to the National Institute of Mental Health (NIMH), an estimated 16 million adults in the United States had at least one major depressive episode in 2012. The World Health Organization (WHO) notes that approximately 350 million people worldwide suffer from depression, a leading cause of disability. I was taught in medical school that depression was a result of a "chemical imbalance" in the brain and that the solution was to correct this with medications.

This theory, which first appeared in a 1965 research article, proposes that a deficiency or underactivity of neurotransmitters (dopamine, serotonin, and norepinephrine) is responsible for depression. This chemical imbalance hypothesis spurred pharmaceutical companies to develop antidepressants known as selective serotonin reuptake inhibitors (SSRIs), but this theory has never been proven. In fact, later research has discredited it. So a whole class of medications and antidepressants were developed based on a false theory. I will explain some of the poor science behind antidepressant medications later on in this chapter and offer some safe and effective natural therapies that can help overcome the effects of depression without harmful side effects.

Table 2: Signs of Depression

Blaming. You focus on other people as the source of your negative feelings, and you refuse to take responsibility for changing yourself: "She's to blame for the way I feel now" or "It's all my parents' fault that I have problems."

Disqualifying the positive. You reject positive experiences by insisting they "don't count" for whatever reason.

(continued)

Table 2: Signs of Depression (*continued*)

Distorted thinking. You see things in black-and-white categories. If your performance falls short of perfect, your see yourself as a total failure.

Emotional reasoning. You assume that your emotions necessarily reflect the way things really are: "I feel it, therefore it must be true."

Fortune-teller error. You anticipate that things will turn out badly, and you feel convinced that your prediction is an already an established fact.

Judgment focus. You view yourself, others, and events in terms of evaluations as good-bad or superior-inferior, rather than simply describing, accepting, or understanding.

Jumping to conclusions. You make a negative interpretation even though there are no definite facts that convincingly support your conclusions.

Mind reading. You arbitrarily conclude that someone is reacting negatively to you, and you don't bother to check this out.

Overgeneralization. You see a single negative event as a never-ending pattern of defeat.

Personalization. You see yourself as the cause of some negative external event that you were not primarily responsible for.

"Should" statements. You try to motivate yourself with "shoulds" and "shouldn'ts." The emotional consequence is guilt. When you direct "should" statements toward others, you feel anger, frustration, and resentment.

Unfair comparisons. You interpret events in terms of standards that are unrealistic. For example, you focus primarily on others who do better than you and find yourself inferior by comparison: "He's more successful than me" or "Others did better than I did on the test."[3]

Why Depression Medications Are Ineffective

An analysis of more than ninety studies failed to show that lowering serotonin levels produced depression in people who were not previously depressed. In fact, in the vast majority of studies, there was no change in the subjects' mood. But perhaps the most compelling argument against the use of the most commonly prescribed antidepressants (SSRIs) is their performance against a placebo. In 2000, researchers studied seven antidepressants (Prozac, Zoloft, Paxil, Effexor, Serzone, Remeron, and Wellbutrin SR), and not one of these blockbuster drugs were found to be significantly more effective in treating depression than a placebo.

In fact, studies found that the antidepressant medications improved the symptoms of depression by 40 percent, while the placebo improved symptoms of depression by 41 percent. Additionally, the older antidepressants, called tricyclics, were found to be 41.7 percent effective in treating the symptoms of depression. In other words, both classes of drugs failed to outperform the placebo. See Table 3 for the adverse side effects of depression medications.[4]

Table 3: Adverse Effects of Depression Meds

You might be surprised to learn what adverse effects are associated with antidepressant medications. According to the *Physician's Desk Reference*, the negative side effects of Prozac include

anorexia

anxiety

depression

drowsiness

esophageal ulceration

headache

heart arrhythmia

insomnia

iver dysfunction

mania

muscle paralysis

pulmonary hypertension

seizures

suicidal ideation[5]

Alternative Treatments for Depression
- **Talk therapy**. In my clinical experience, psychotherapy has been shown to be an extremely effective treatment for depression without the risk of adverse side effects associated with medications. Finding the right therapist can take some time, but in my opinion, it's well worth the effort, so don't rush to the pill bottle before giving it a try.

- **Exercise.** Countless studies have shown conclusively that people who boost their heart rates through exercise also lower their risk of depression and anxiety. Why does moving help keep us happy and calm? One reason is that increased blood flow releases feel-good neurotransmitters, including endorphins, or "endogenous morphine" (you read that correctly)—the brain's natural opioids that produce feelings of euphoria and well-being. Simply put, the more you exercise, the better you will feel mentally.

  The good news for exercise haters is that you don't have to run a marathon (or even break a sweat—though it's good if you do) to get a brain buzz. Research has shown that as little as twenty minutes of walking can do the trick. One Norwegian survey published in 2013 found that those who engaged in any kind of exercise, even a small amount, reported improved mental health compared with people who, despite the alluring Scandinavian mountains and fjords, chose a sedentary lifestyle.[6]

- **Food and mood.** Have you ever come back after lunch and felt tired, nauseous, or a little "foggy"? The reason for this is that your enteric or gut nervous system might be reacting to something you ate and is sending signals to your brain. Our central nervous system and gut are wired to react to certain foods, so you should avoid SAD foods that will make you feel depressed. The best prescription for preventing and treating depression might be to clean up your gut and eat a healthy diet of fresh fruits and vegetables and whole, unrefined grains. In addition, drink adequate amounts of water for your weight; avoid artificial sweeteners such Nutrasweet and Splenda, which can disrupt the body's production of serotonin as well as cause problems with gut bacteria; and consume sufficient amounts of unrefined salt.

- **Clear up your allergies**. As I mentioned in the previous chapter, I have seen a relationship between food allergies and depression in my patients. An allergy to gluten, for example, is commonly related to depression. Likewise, I've also found sugar and dairy allergies in many depressed patients I've treated. An allergy to sugar can manifest as changes in blood sugar levels, leading to hypoglycemic episodes, and the use of antibiotics and hormones in conventionally raised cows can further exacerbate anxiety. (For more on this, read my *Guide to a Dairy-Free Diet*.)

- **Light therapy**. In addition to SAD foods, there is another kind of SAD called seasonal affective disorder. I have seen a number of patients with this condition, especially during the winter months. The low level of sunlight during winter, resulting in lowered serotonin and vitamin D, gives rise to more frequent bouts of depression. Using antidepressants to treat SAD will only target the symptom and not the underlying cause of the depression—a lack of sunlight.

- **An imbalanced hormonal system**. I have seen countless patients become depressed from suffering with a hormonal system in disarray. This can include hormones from the thyroid, adrenals, brain, and sex glands. When the underlying imbalanced hormonal system is corrected with the use of bioidentical natural hormones, with great frequency, my experience has shown that depression and other mood disorders either significantly improve or resolve.

- **Tryptophan increases serotonin levels**. The body can convert the amino acid tryptophan into serotonin, which can cross the blood-brain barrier (the semipermeable membrane that separates the circulating blood from the brain's fluid in the central nervous system) and facilitate the production of serotonin. I recommend getting tryptophan in high-protein food, such as organically or wild-raised animals—do not eat meat from animals raised in factory farms that are fed corn or soy, and worse, are inhumanely treated. Organic farmers that raise their animals with grasses and other plants that were meant to eaten are a far healthier choice. These foods include beef, chicken, dairy products, eggs, pork, turkey, and venison.

- **Correct adrenal and hormonal imbalances**. Studies show that when the gut gets inflamed, so does the brain. The consequences include depression, anxiety, and a host of other mental and brain health issues, including ADD and attention deficit hyperactive disorder (ADHD). Because the gut microbiome plays a key role in regulating everything from digestion and metabolism to immune function, it stands to reason that the gut-brain connection can also affect our mood. Depression is brought on in people who have LGS due to a poor diet and nutrient deficiency. As you become nutrient depleted, many things in the body lose their homeostatic balance, including the neurological system. When your neurotransmitters are out of whack or your adrenal and thyroid hormones are imbalanced, you must get the proper nutrients or hormones to correct the imbalances.

Maria's Story

Maria, who is in her sixties and works at a bank, came to me pleading for help. She was depressed and not getting much joy out of life. She was also anxious at work and told me, "I don't want to go on living like this!" Upon examination, I found that she had multiple gut issues, including discomfort after eating and sluggish bowels. She had gained weight, which made her even unhappier. She was also having trouble thinking clearly and couldn't recall names.

She had been to many doctors about her IBS and depression. They prescribed medications to treat both, including antidepressants, which gave her no relief. She said the antidepressants simply made her feel tired, so she stopped taking them.

In my examination, I asked her about her eating habits, which was a standard American diet of refined salt, sugar, and oils; lots of dairy through sweetened yogurt; and many carbohydrates with oatmeal for breakfast, bread during the day, and pasta followed by sweets at night. She wasn't drinking enough water, but she was having six to eight cups of coffee a day with a little bit of juice. She looked pale and had dry skin, a dry tongue, and dry eyes. I noticed vertical ridges on her nails—all signs of dehydration. Her stomach was tender to the touch, and she was only having two bowel movements a week with the help of laxatives.

I told her to clean up her diet to go on a Paleo regimen—more protein and whole foods—to avoid all refined foods, and to drink half her body weight in water. Her gut and brain could not feel better when she was dehydrated because 75 percent of the brain consists of water.

I did a stool test to look at her flora and bloodwork to evaluate her hormonal and nutritional status. After making the dietary changes, she said she had more energy, her head was clearer, and she began having more normal bowel movements, though they were still sluggish. . . . Her stool analysis came back showing low amounts of good bacteria, an overgrowth of bad bacteria (candida), and antibodies to casein from the dairy. She was also deficient in vitamin B12 and magnesium, and she was hypothyroid. At that visit, I put her on B12 shots (1 mg, twice a week) and told her to take small amounts of iodine for her thyroid. I also gave her 200 mg of magnesium, oregano oil supplements, and a two-week course of an antiyeast medication. I told her to exercise twenty to thirty minutes a day (walking was fine). Furthermore, I placed her on a pre- and probiotic regimen to supply her gut with the right nutrients and bacteria to replenish it.

I saw her two months later, and she said she felt almost completely better. All her symptoms disappeared, including her depression and foggy brain. She was still struggling a bit with her diet, but I promised that if she continued to make these changes, she would be better, which proved to be true.

Attention Deficit Disorder and Attention Deficit Hyperactivity Disorder

As of 2011, the Centers for Disease Control and Prevention (CDC) estimated that approximately 11 percent of US children ages four to seventeen (6.4 million) have been diagnosed with ADHD. The percentage of children given an ADHD diagnosis continued to rise, from 7.8 percent in 2003 to 11 percent in 2011. Most families are given one option—take medication such as Ritalin or Adderall, both stimulants. It's understandable why many concerned parents would try them, feeling the pressure from conventional doctors or teachers who don't want disrupted classrooms. But the fact is, there are insufficient data to prove that ADHD medications are safe for the long term, and there is some evidence suggesting that drugs like Adderall can be addictive and even produce suicidal thoughts in some patients.

In contrast, research to support dietary approaches to ADHD dates back more than forty years. Dr. Ben Feingold, a pioneer in the area of nutrition and behavior, studied how certain foods and chemicals affected behavior back in the sixties. According to Dr. Feingold, "Hyperactivity can be triggered by synthetic additives, specifically synthetic colors, synthetic flavors and the preservatives BHA, BHT (and TBHQ added later), and also a group of foods containing a natural salicylate radical." He believed that "any compound, natural or synthetic, can induce an adverse reaction if the individual has the appropriate genetic profile."

Leaky Gut and ADD/ADHD

When a child has a problem with focus or attention, we naturally assume there is an issue in the brain. And while there generally is an imbalance of neurotransmitters, what if the problem stemmed from a leaky gut? A leaky gut could explain why certain foods, dyes, vaccines, and other chemicals can affect some children with attention disorders, while others seem to be relatively unscathed. Although nutritional approaches do not work for everyone, studies have found that a high percentage of ADD/ADHD patients respond to nutritional changes.

According to a Dutch study published in a 2011 issue of *Lancet*, 64 percent of diagnosed cases of ADHD were caused by a hypersensitivity to food (see Table 4); when the food was removed, the symptoms improved. Says lead author Dr. Lidy

Pelsser, "We have good news—that food is the main cause of ADHD. We've got bad news too—that we have to train physicians to monitor this procedure because it cannot be done by a physician who is not trained."

Table 4: The Three Most Common Foods Associated with ADHD Symptoms

---

Dairy. According to Doris Rapp, MD, author of *Is This Your Child?*, diary is at the top of the list of foods that cause behavior, focus, and attention problems. Other signs that your child could have a problem with dairy include bedwetting (past toddlerhood); asthma; temper tantrums; frequent ear, upper respiratory, or sinus infections; and vocal tics or throat clearing.

Wheat/gluten. According to the book *Dangerous Grains* by James Braly, MD, and Ron Hoggan, MA, "about 70 percent of children with untreated celiac disease show exactly the same abnormalities in brain-wave patterns as those who have been diagnosed with attention deficit disorder." Mood disorders are also common with gluten intolerances—including aggressive, angry, bullying, and irritable behavior.

Food colorings and additives. A total of fifteen million pounds of dyes are added to foods each year, many of which are directly marketed at schoolchildren. As Dr. Feingold found as early as the sixties, food dyes have been linked to behavioral problems, hyperactivity, allergic reactions, and even some cancers. A study published in a 2007 issue of *Lancet* concluded that food dyes increased hyperactivity in children. Based on this study, the British government banned the use of food dyes, and all foods that contain dyes in Europe must come with a warning label that says, "May have an adverse effect on activity and attention in children."

Unfortunately, parents of kids with ADHD are rarely told about nutritional/supplementary options. I submit that if the root cause of the problem is food sensitivities, shouldn't we start by treating the attention and behavior issues by identifying and eliminating any offending foods and, if needed, adding nutritional supplements? Parents can look for a practitioner who can help them navigate this approach to treating focus and attention issues. The Netherlands study shows that a significant number of kids might just benefit from nutritional changes. I realize that a food elimination diet it is not as easy as popping a pill every day, but it treats the underlying cause of the illness, and even those who end up taking medications might also benefit from trying a nutritional approach to treating these disorders.[7]

These are three of the most common things to watch out for when it comes to ADHD, but there are other foods/substances that could be causing focus and attention problems, including high-fructose corn syrup/sugar, grains, soy, eggs, and corn.

Table 5: Common Nutrient Deficiencies in Kids with ADHD

When you have LGS, you are at risk of consuming foods that the body is sensitive to, which can damage to the small intestine and lead to poor nutrient absorption. Another reason for nutrient deficiencies is eating a standard American diet that is lacking in macro- and micronutrients. The following are some of the most common nutrient deficiencies associated with ADHD:

Omega-3 fatty acids. The brain is composed of more than 60 percent fat, so diets must have sufficient amounts of healthy fats in order for our brain to function well. Omega-3 and omega-6 fatty acids are known as essential fats, since we cannot manufacture them and we must get them in our diet or we will die. Both fats are essential for brain function. A 1996 Purdue University study revealed that kids with learning and behavior problems had lower levels of omega-3 in their blood. Omega-3s can be found in fish like salmon, tuna, and sardines, as well as nuts, seeds like chia, and fish oils. Omega-6 fats can be found in many foods, including free-range animal products and healthy oils.

(continued)

B vitamins. Known as the antistress vitamins, B vitamins are important for regulating our energy, sleep cycles, and metabolism. They are also needed to create neurotransmitters. Because B vitamins are water soluble, they are not stored in our bodies for very long, so they can become easily depleted, and deficiency is very common. Vitamin B6 (synthesizes dopamine, serotonin, and norepinephrine) and vitamin B12 (synthesizes amino acids that promote concentration) are important for brain function.

Vitamin B6 with magnesium decreases central nervous system hyperactivity. I have been checking vitamin B12 levels in every patient that sees me for the last twenty years. I would estimate that more than one-third of the patients I've tested are low in B12. A B12 deficiency can cause children to be hyperactive and anxious and can also cause obsessive behavior. If severe enough, it can lead to pernicious anemia and serious neurological issues. Vitamin B12 can only be found in animal products, and B12 deficiency is common in people with food sensitivities or digestive issues, as its digestion and absorption is complicated. So identifying food sensitivities and removing them is a crucial part of treatment. More information on vitamin B12 can be found in my book *Vitamin B12 for Health*.

Magnesium. It is estimated that up to 95 percent of kids with ADHD might be deficient in magnesium. Magnesium is known as the "calming mineral," and studies show that supplementing with magnesium can reduce hyperactivity in kids. The fourth most abundant mineral in the body, magnesium plays a key role in building strong bones, facilitating nerve functions, regulating blood pressure, maintaining body temperature, and allowing muscles (including the heart) to reach a state of relaxation. Magnesium also helps calcium get into the bones by synthesizing vitamin D. In addition to ADHD/hyperactivity, low magnesium levels can be associated with constipation, restless leg syndrome, sleep issues, migraines, foot or eye twitches, muscle cramps/pain, irritability, and even an elevated risk of heart disease/stroke.

(continued)

**Table 5: Common Nutrient Deficiencies
in Kids with ADHD** (*continued*)

Zinc. Low zinc can lead to slow growth, delayed puberty, and attention issues. Taking ADHD medication can also deplete zinc levels. A study published in 2011 in the *Journal of Child and Adolescent Psychopharmacology* found that those receiving a zinc supplement required 37 percent less amphetamine to get the same results compared to those taking amphetamine plus placebo. The zinc appeared to improve the effectiveness of the amphetamine so that a lower dose was needed for desired results.[8]

Meghan's Story

Meghan was eight and having trouble in school. She was unable to concentrate, and teachers were complaining that she wasn't doing well in class or on her assignments. Meghan also complained of frequent stomachaches. She said her stomach hurt all the time and it never felt right. Her parents, who were concerned, took her to a doctor who diagnosed her with ADHD and put her on Ritalin. They read up on the drug and became concerned, so they came to me looking for an alternative.

On my exam, I felt that Meghan was suffering from LGS. I did a dietary history and found that she was getting a lot of sugar due to her sweet tooth—having lots of candy and other desserts. Her school lunches consisted of lots of pizza and pasta, and she drink juice instead of water. Like many children, she was a finicky eater, and she eschewed fruits and veggies.

Caveat: Although Vitamin B6 is water soluble, it is the one B vitamin that can accumulate in the body and possibly lead to permanent nerve damage if taken in high doses for long period of time. Always consult a doctor when taking this supplement.

Otherwise she was in good health, but she wasn't happy about how she was feeling. She couldn't explain why. I talked to her about her diet and explained that she was eating things that were making her sick.

So her parents cleaned up the fridge and the pantry and threw away everything that had refined sugar in it. They packed a lunch box with a water bottle instead of having her eat the prepared school lunch. They stopped buying juice. I did bloodwork on her that showed common nutritional deficiencies such as low vitamin C, low B vitamins (particularly B12 and thiamine), and low essential minerals (found through hair testing). I put her on a good multivitamin to correct this nutritional imbalance.

When I saw her again in a few months, her concentration had improved, her grades had improved, and she said she felt happier. And her gut symptoms were much improved. Her mother said that daily stomachaches were a thing of the past, and now she only complained about her stomach when she ate bad food. The parents continued to make her lunch, which now included fruits and vegetables. She made a full recovery with the use of stimulant medications. She is still fine five years later. As a young teenager, she now lectures her fellow students about nutrition and tells me she wants to be a doctor.

Headaches

There are many causes of headaches, including hypothyroidism, hyperthyroidism, drugs, nutrient deficiencies, or inflammation of the brain. The best treatment for headaches is drinking more water. Again, because the brain is 75 percent water, it is essential to help the brain function properly.

When the brain becomes dehydrated, the brain's receptors become more active. I've treated hundreds of patients with headaches over the years just by giving them more water, and their headaches either decreased in frequency or went away entirely.

Dietary triggers can bring on headaches in certain people. Keep a log of the foods you have eaten before a headache or migraine attack and see whether the removal of these foods from your diet reduces or eliminates your headaches. For a list of foods that might trigger headaches, go to the National Headache Foundation's website at http://www.headaches .org/headache-sufferers-diet/.

Diane's Story

Diane, who was in her forties, was having daily headaches and migraines every few weeks. They varied in intensity, and stress made them worse. She got some relief from Motrin, Advil, and ibuprofen, but such medications gave her stomach problems, including bloating. She'd been to neurologists and internists who tried different medications on her, but nothing helped. She would go to bed with a headache and wake up with a headache.

All the while, she also suffered with stomachaches and bloating. When I examined her, I found stomach tenderness from LGS that caused alternating constipation and diarrhea. I asked how much water she drank, and she said hardly any. Instead, she drank coffee, soda, and juice. Her skin and tongue were dry, and she had vertical ridges on her nails from severe dehydration. I advised her to drink half her body weight in water daily and cut back on the anti-inflammatory medications. (Anti-inflammatory medications are a common cause of LGS, as they can irritate the gut lining causing inflammation and leakiness.) She also cut out all refined sugars and carbs from her diet.

When I saw her again in a month, she gave me a big hug. She said it took nine days, but on that ninth day she woke up without a headache. Gradually over the next few weeks, her headaches went away completely. She was thinking and feeling better, and her energy was up. Her gut was also feeling better; the inflammation was gone. She said she learned that what you eat can affect the way you feel and that medications aren't always the answer.

Dementia

Dementia is the umbrella term for the loss of cognitive function, such as reasoning and memory, that is severe enough to interfere with daily life. There are many types of dementia, including Alzheimer's disease, a neurodegenerative disease that involves the loss or dying off of brain cells over time. Other lesser-known neurodegenerative diseases that cause dementia include Lewy body dementia and Pick's disease. Dementia can be caused by a series of strokes, alcohol and drug abuse, or head trauma (either a single injury or multiple blows), as well as infections such as AIDS.

According to a 2000 report from the WHO, approximately 6 to 10 percent of the population sixty-five years of age and older in North America have dementia, with Alzheimer's accounting for two-thirds of those cases. Sadly, there is no cure of Alzheimer's at the time of this writing. There are medications available that help treat the symptoms, but they have only a marginal benefit and do not prevent the progression of the disease—yet another reason we must do everything in our power to see to it that our brain stays healthy and fit for as long as possible!

One of the things I tell my concerned patients is that there are countless treatable conditions that might be causing or contributing to their memory lapses, such as vitamin deficiency or a hormonal imbalance. Again, many of the conditions that masquerade as dementia are reversible. I also reassure my patients that certain changes in brain function are simply a normal part of living longer. As we get older, the speed at which we process information slows down, and our memory might not be as strong as when we were younger. As frustrating as this can be (like forgetting where you put your keys or the name of an old friend), there are aspects of the brain that actually improve with age, such as our ability to make wise decisions.

When I suspect that my patients are having memory problems due to an unhealthy lifestyle, which is treatable or early onset Alzheimer's disease, my approach is the same. I take a thorough medical history, including a dietary history, as well as a blood work-up, an evaluation of past health problems, and a review of their medical record. I find out what medications and supplements they are taking and review their dietary and family history. I ask about their lifestyle choices, including personal habits and social life.

I might suggest a stool analysis or a neurological exam, such as magnetic resonance imaging (MRI) or computerized tomography (CT) scans. The results will often provide more information about the underlying cause of their symptoms. Whatever the diagnosis—whether it's Alzheimer's, depression masquerading as dementia, or simply sleep deprivation—we sit down and carefully go over the next steps we need to take to ensure that their brain is functioning at its best.[9]

Ray's Story

Ray was a sixty-eight-year-old business executive who was extremely successful. His wife was a patient of mine for years, and she asked me to examine him because she became worried that something was happening to him mentally. He used keep the books for this business but gave them to her to do because he couldn't do the math anymore. I asked him if he felt there was something going on with his brain, and he said he was starting to worry because he wasn't able to do the simple mental functions that he could do before.

After taking a dietary history, I found that Ray was eating a standard American diet. He didn't drink any water (he had sodas instead) and ate a lot of dairy and gluten. He had multiple nutritional deficiencies and dehydration. He was an active man who ran every day, but it was becoming increasingly difficult. He stopped getting that runner's high he used to. He started having constipation and would go only once a week. He took fiber supplements, but he still had constipation and diarrhea.

A neurologist diagnosed him with Lewy body disease, which is a horrific disease like accelerated Alzheimer's disease. He gave him six months to a year to live. He offered some medications that might slow down the disease, but there is no cure. When I saw him after the bloodwork, I found antibodies to gluten and dairy that caused inflammation in his gut, leading to LGS and an inflamed brain. I told him he wouldn't get better unless he cut out the dairy and grains and went on a gluten-free diet. I put him on a ketosis diet, which is eating only fat and protein—no carbohydrates. When you stop eating carbs, you break down the fat into ketone bodies, and the brain cells produce energy out of glucose and fat.

I felt his brain wasn't processing glucose properly, so he needed and alternative resource. A stool test revealed candida overgrowth. He needed to stop eating all foods that turned into sugar and to drink water. He was low on vitamin B12, thiamine, zinc, and iodine and hypothyroid. I told him that if he didn't change his diet, he would die in a year. He listened, and his leaky gut and other symptoms went away. We treated the candida with oregano oil, grapefruit seed extract, and a short course of nystatin, which is used to treat yeast infections in the stomach.

When he and his wife came to see me next, she started crying. She gave me a big hug and thanked me because her husband had "come back to life." She said, "You saved his life—he was dying in front of me." He had 40 percent brain function when I saw him, and he returned to about 90 percent brain function. Whenever he strayed from his diet, his dementia would return, and although he was fine for nearly four more years, this story does not have a happy ending. Ray returned to his old eating habits and finally succumbed to the disease. I am convinced that had he continued to be vigilant with his dietary treatment program, he might be alive today.

Alzheimer's Disease

A 2015 study was published in the journal *Nature* about how changes in the gut microbiome might produce a higher risk of Alzheimer's. This study found that common industrial ingredients known as emulsifiers (chemicals used to improve food's texture and increase shelf life) is associated with abnormal inflammation of the digestive tract. There has been a dramatic increase in Alzheimer's disease since the widespread adoption of chemical food additives. Similarly, other research has found a link between disrupted gut microbiomes and the development of Parkinson's disease and autism (see page 188).[10]

Ten Warning Signs of Early Onset Dementia from the Alzheimer's Association

If you or a loved one notice any of the following warning signs, please make note of your concerns by writing on another sheet of paper or on your device, and take it with you to your doctor. This list was provided by the Alzheimer's Association (http://www.alz.org).

1. **Memory loss that disrupts daily life**. One of the most common signs of Alzheimer's, especially in the early stages, is forgetting recent events or newly learned information (short-term memory loss). Others include forgetting important names, dates, or events (but often recalling them later on); repeatedly asking for the same information; dependence on memory aides (e.g., reminder notes); or asking family members to do things that you used to handle on your own.

2. **Challenges in planning or solving problems**. Some people might experience changes in their ability to develop and follow a plan or work with numbers. You might have trouble following a familiar recipe or keeping track of monthly bills. You might have difficulty concentrating and take much longer to do things than you did before. A typical example is making occasional errors when balancing a checkbook.

3. **Difficulty completing familiar tasks at home, at work, or at leisure**. People with Alzheimer's often find it hard to complete daily tasks. Sometimes people get lost when driving to a familiar location or have trouble managing a budget at work or remembering the rules of a favorite game. Sometimes you might require help using the settings on the microwave or recording a television show (something you've done countless times in the past).

4. **Confusion with time or place**. People with Alzheimer's can lose track of dates, seasons, and the passage of time. They might have trouble understanding something if it is not happening immediately. Sometimes they might forget where they are or how they got there. You or a loved one might get confused, for example, about what day of the week it is before figuring it out later.

5. **Trouble understanding visual images and spatial relationships**. For some people, having vision problems is a sign of Alzheimer's. They might have difficulty reading, judging distance, and determining color or contrast. This perception problem might include not recognizing their own reflection in a mirror. Check with your doctor to determine if these vision changes due to cataracts.

6. **New problems with words in speaking or writing**. People with Alzheimer's might have trouble following or joining a conversation or finding the right word. They might stop in the middle of a conversation and have no idea how to continue, or they might repeat themselves. They can struggle with vocabulary, have difficulty finding the right word, or call things by the wrong name (e.g., calling a watch a "hand clock").

7. **Misplacing things and losing the ability to retrace steps**. A person with Alzheimer's disease might put things in unusual places. They might lose things and not be able to retrace their steps to find them again. In severe cases, they might accuse others of stealing. This can occur as the disease progresses. Misplacing things from time to time, such as a pair of glasses or the remote control, is not something to be concerned about (we all do this every once in a while).

8. **Decreased or poor judgment**. People with Alzheimer's might experience changes in judgment or decision making. They might use poor judgment when dealing with money, for example, such as falling victim to pernicious telemarketers. They might also pay less attention to grooming or keeping themselves clean. Making an occasional bad decision is not reason for concern, but if this behavior continues, it's a red flag.

9. **Withdrawal from work or social activities**. People with Alzheimer's might stop engaging in hobbies, social activities, work projects, or sports they once enjoyed. They might have trouble keeping up with a favorite sports team, for example. They might also start to withdraw from others. Simply feeling weary of work, family, or social obligations is not unusual, however.

10. **Changes in mood and personality**. The mood and personalities of people with Alzheimer's can change dramatically. They can suddenly become confused, suspicious, depressed, fearful, or anxious. They might become easily upset, especially when they are out of their comfort zone, or irritable when a routine is disrupted.

If you have questions about any of these warning signs, the Alzheimer's Association recommends consulting a physician. Early diagnosis provides the best opportunities for treatment, support, and future planning. For more information, go to http://www.alz.org or call 800-272-3900.

Alternative Treatment for Alzheimer's and Dementia

A growing number of herbal remedies, dietary supplements, and "medical foods" are promoted as memory enhancers or treatments to delay or prevent Alzheimer's disease and related dementias. Claims about the safety and effectiveness of these products, however, are based largely on testimonials, anecdotal evidence, and a small body of scientific research, so consult with a medical practitioner you trust before choosing an alternative treatment.

Here are some recommendations from the Alzheimer's Association.[11]

Omega-3 Fatty Acids

You have already read about omega-3s in this book, which are a type of polyunsaturated fatty acid (PUFA). Research has linked certain types of omega-3s to a reduced risk of heart disease and stroke. The US Food and Drug Administration (FDA) permits supplements and foods to display labels with "a qualified health claim" for two omega-3s called docosahexaenoic acid (DHA) and eicosapentaenoic acid (EPA). The labels may state, "Supportive but not conclusive research shows that consumption of EPA and DHA omega-3 fatty acids may reduce the risk of coronary heart disease" and then list the amount of DHA or EPA in the product. The FDA recommends taking no more than a combined total of 3 grams of DHA or EPA a day, with no more than 2 grams from supplements.

Research has also linked high intake of omega-3s to a possible reduction in risk of dementia or cognitive decline. The chief omega-3 in the brain is DHA, which is found in the fatty membranes that surround nerve cells, especially at the microscopic junctions where cells connect to one another. Theories about why omega-3s might influence dementia risk include their benefit for the heart and blood vessels, anti-inflammatory effects, and support and protection of nerve cell membranes.

Two studies reported at the 2009 Alzheimer's Association International Conference on Alzheimer's Disease found mixed results for the possible benefits of DHA:

- The first study was a large federally funded clinical trial conducted by the Alzheimer's Disease Cooperative Study (ADCS). In the ADCS study, participants with mild to moderate Alzheimer's disease taking 2 grams of DHA daily fared no better overall than those who took a placebo. The data indicated preliminary but not conclusive evidence that participants without the Alzheimer's risk gene (APOE-e4) might have experienced a slight benefit. More research is needed to confirm whether that preliminary finding is valid. You can read the results of this study in the November 3, 2010, issue of the *Journal of the American Medical Association*.[12]
- The second study—Memory Improvement with DHA (MIDAS)—enrolled older adults with normal age-related cognitive decline. Those who took 900 mg of DHA daily scored slightly better on a computerized memory test than those receiving the placebo. MIDAS was conducted by Martek Biosciences, the manufacturer of the DHA used in both studies.

Experts agree that more research is needed and that there is not yet sufficient evidence to recommend DHA or any other omega-3 fatty acids to treat or prevent Alzheimer's disease. And omega-3 fatty acids need to be taken in balance with omega-6 fatty acids.

LGS Link to Alzheimer's and Autism

A 2015 study published in the journal *Nature* found another mechanism by which gut microbes might influence human physiology. That study showed that the common industrial food ingredients known as emulsifiers (chemicals used to improve food's texture and have a longer shelf life) produce changes in the gut microbiome that lead to more of the inflammation associated with inflammatory bowel disease (IBD) and metabolic syndrome.

Metabolic syndrome is a cluster of physiological symptoms linked with a higher risk of heart disease, diabetes, liver disease, and Alzheimer's disease. It's associated with high levels of systemic inflammation. IBD is characterized by abnormal inflammation of the digestive tract. Both conditions have dramatically increased since the widespread use of chemical food additives. Other studies have linked a disrupted microbiome with the development of autism.[13]

Autism and Leaky Gut

Tim Buie, MD, assistant professor at Harvard Medical School and pediatric gastroenterologist at the Lurie Center for Autism at Massachusetts General Hospital for children, gave a recent talk on "Gastrointestinal Problems in Autism and the Brain-Gut Connection." The following is excerpt:

> The prevalence of autism, as most of us know, has been on the rise. When I graduated from medical school in 1984, it was one in 5,000 individuals. . . . The current prevalence of autism is about one in 68 individuals, according to the CDC. No one has had a really good explanation for the increase.
>
> We do know that, in terms of gastrointestinal issues, the frequency of GI problems seems to be a good deal higher than the general pediatric population. We did a consensus study of the literature back in 2010, published in the *Journal of Pediatrics*, that talked about the kinds of presentations that [autistic] children have, including acid reflux and constipation. A more recent paper by Dr. Barbara McElhanon at Emory University reported that there is about a 3.2 times higher frequency of these gastrointestinal issues in autistic children than the general pediatric patient population. According to these studies, somewhere between about 50 percent and 70 percent of kids with autism will have chronic gastrointestinal symptoms as well. People have reported symptoms consistent with acid reflux, and increased leaky gut syndrome has been described in a number of studies.
>
> The finding of leaky gut in particular has been somewhat inconsistent partly because the testing for intestinal permeability is really quite poor. And doctors who do this work haven't been able to show a well-done standard of what accounts for increased intestinal permeability. We do a number of studies

where we give a nonabsorbable sugar and we measure for that sugar in the urine to see if it has leaked across the gut lining. But it hasn't been reliable even from the same individual at different times to really help us know how many of these kids have this increased permeability.

But this is important because if the permeability of the gut is disrupted it's probably how we sensitize to food proteins and develop food allergy. And so, if there's a problem with digestion or there's a problem with inflammation, there may be increased permeability as a result, which may be why we're seeing a higher frequency of food allergy or other issues in this population. And we know from work that's done at the UC Davis MIND Institute [the Medical Investigation of Neurodevelopmental Disorders is an international research center for neurodevelopmental disorders], among other places, that there are altered immune responses in the gut of children with autism.

Children with autism have a right to a medical work-up, and . . . it's important to really consider these underlying medical conditions that may be making behavior of children with autism worse or their focus worse so that they can not make progress. We suggest that these children really need a dietitian to evaluate them and make sure that they don't have evidence of dietary insufficiency that might be accounting for some of these problems.[14]

Next, learn what foods are best to heal your LGS symptoms and illnesses.

The Healthy Gut Diet

Energy is about more than fueling your body—a higher kind of energy comes from the joy of eating.

—Deepak Chopra

Eat a Real Meal

If you are like many Americans who eat a typical Western diet, I hope you are now motivated to turn over a new leaf (maybe some dark green ones) and make the necessary dietary changes that will heal your gut and resolve whatever chronic condition or disease you might be suffering from. Understanding how to shore up a leaky gut and the role that bacteria and other microbes living in your intestinal tract play is a good long-term investment in your health and well-being. As the previous chapters have demonstrated, there is mounting evidence that a healthful diet with an array of good intestinal microbiota helps us process nutrients and bolsters our immune system.

By contrast, eating an unhealthy diet will have consequences that extend far beyond a belly ache; it might put you at risk for developing everything from allergies and inflammation, cancer, and diabetes and obesity, to mental health conditions like depression and attention deficit hyperactive disorder (ADHD). Changing your diet (and microbiome) might not happen overnight, but if you follow the advice in this chapter, the payoff is enormous—namely, more time to enjoy a good-quality life.

Keep in mind that all guts are not created equal. Your intestinal ecosystem started when you were born and has continued to evolve as you age. It is influenced by way you've been eating and living (e.g., if you have been smoking, drinking too much alcohol, or lacking in sleep and exercise), stress, and other factors that determine how you process nutrients. If your diet consists of cheeseburgers and pepperoni pizza, your gut will not be healthy. A healthy diet consisting of fruits, vegetables, and unprocessed food, however, builds a stronger foundation of more varied microbiota. The good news is that it's never too late to start eating a healthy diet, which includes eating fresh, locally grown whole, unprocessed foods that do not contain hormones or pesticides.

One of the questions I get most often from my patients is, "What should I eat?" I will answer that question and more and tell you how to heal your leaky gut and cultivate an even healthier one by eliminating the foods that are making you sick.

Don't Be a Belly Flop

One reason Americans do not eat as well as they should is misinformation. Conventional organizations such as the American Diabetic Association (ADA) and the American Medical Association (AMA) parrot the same advice: "Follow the food pyramid."

Unfortunately, following the food pyramid ensures that your diet will consist of too many refined, nutrient-depleted foods. But my experience as a holistic physician has clearly shown that a diet of healthy food containing vitamins, minerals, enzymes, and other healing agents for our bodies is the best choice because it leads to enhanced immune systems and overall good health. Refined food—including refined sugar, salt, oils, and grains that is in so much of what we eat—is, by definition, nutritionally depleted. These foods are abundantly available on in our supermarkets because they are inexpensive to make, and they are loaded with preservatives so they will last longer. *Ca-ching* for food manufacturers. A belly flop for the consumer.

The Twinkie Defense

Sorry, Hostess lovers, but there is no defending the Twinkie, that spongy yellow cake filled with white faux frosting and unpronounceable ingredients. It has become an iconic symbol of processed foods because urban legend has it that it is the roach of snack foods (i.e., it cannot be destroyed). The truth is somewhat less dramatic but nonetheless terrifying: a Twinkie has a shelf life of forty-five days. (Compare that to a homemade cake made of eggs, flour, and butter left uncovered at room temperature, which will last only four to five days.) It was the subject of the book *Twinkie, Deconstructed* by Steve Ettlinger.

A Twinkie is a highly processed food with no less than three dozen or so ingredients such as the yummy-sounding sodium stearoyl lactylate and others that come from a lab. Unfortunately, this is typical of thousands of other processed food products out there. Why would manufacturers knowingly put these unsavory chemicals into a product that both children and adults readily consume? Butter and eggs spoil, so food companies cleverly devised a way to defy the laws of nature. The Twinkie's butter flavor, Ettlinger says, comes from diacetyl, the same compound used in microwave popcorn (another processed food that should be taken off the market, in my opinion).

Instead of eggs, Twinkies have polysorbate 60, an emulsifier made from corn syrup and ethylene oxide (which, according to Ettlinger, is "derived from an oil well"—thank you, Exxon). With polysorbate 60, he told an NPR reporter, "You can get this wonderful goo that resembles egg yolk, only more powerful." The combination of these ingredients extends the Twinkie's shelf life. Still want to put these plastic-wrapped treats into your children's lunch boxes?[1]

Now for a deconstruction of the foods that many of us eat—the good and the bad.

What Are Carbohydrates?

Carbohydrates provide quick fuel for the body in the form of sugars, starches, and fiber. They are found mostly in plant foods, such as fruits, vegetables, grains, and potatoes. Milk also contains some carbs. Carbohydrates are sugars that come in two main forms—simple and complex, which are also referred to as simple sugars and starches, respectively. The difference between a simple and complex carb is in how fast it is digested and absorbed and its chemical structure.

Simple carbs (e.g., sucrose, or table sugar, and fructose from fruit) are very sweet to the taste and are digested quickly by the body. Complex carbs are pleasant to the taste, but they are not as sweet as simple carbs and take longer to digest (see Table 1).

Table 1: Simple versus Complex Carbohydrates

Simple
Fructose: fruit, honey, high fructose corn syrup
Glucose: dextrose, corn syrup
Lactose: milk, dairy
Sucrose: table sugar, brown sugar

Complex
Fiber: whole wheat, breads, cereals, oats, legumes, psyllium, rice bran, barley
Starches: flour, bread, rice, oats, barley, potatoes, legumes, vegetables

Which Carbohydrates Should You Avoid?

Like cholesterol and bacteria, there are good and bad carbohydrates. Unrefined carbohydrates, which are full of minerals, vitamins, enzymes, and fiber, are a healthy food choice. Unrefined carbohydrates contain naturally occurring sugars found in many food products such as fruits and vegetables. Refined carbs, on the other hand, contain little or no nutrients and are not healthy for our bodies. Avoid refined carbohydrates in the form of white sugar, soft drinks, and candy that give you plenty of calories but little or no nutrients.

How Are Carbs Refined?

The process of refining carbohydrates entails taking out all the healthy nutrients (e.g., vitamins, minerals, enzymes) and leaving only the sugar molecules. As I explained earlier, the food industry refines its products to extend shelf life. Once healthy nutrients are removed from the food, there is nothing that can spoil, so it can sit on a shelf forever. Because there is no expiration date on a refined product, it's cheaper compared to a whole food (unrefined) that has an expiration date. Eating too much refined food can speed up our expiration dates as well!

How to Tell If a Product Is Refined

Anything in a package that has no expiration date is refined. White flour, white sugar, high-fructose corn syrup, white pasta, and white rice are common refined carbohydrates.

What Effect Do Carbohydrates Have on Blood Sugar in the Body?

Our bodies turn simple, or refined, carbohydrates into glucose (sugar) quickly. Eating too many refined carbs can mess up your blood sugar regulation. The refined sugars in candy and soft drinks, for example, and refined grains in white flour and white rice, cause blood sugar levels to spike more quickly than a whole-food product. This could increase your risk of developing health problems, including hormonal imbalances and diabetes. Unrefined carbohydrates such as whole grains are broken down more slowly, allowing blood sugar to rise gradually.

What Is the Glycemic Index?

The glycemic index (see Table 2) was developed to measure how quickly carbohydrates enter the bloodstream as glucose. To keep blood sugar from rising, I recommend that you eat foods with a low glycemic index of less than 50 percent. Another way to keep blood sugar from rising is to eat carbohydrates along with whole foods that contain protein, fat, and other nutrients that help slow the entry of sugar into the body. For example, if you are going to eat bread or rice, combine it with a lean protein or vegetables.

Table 2: Glycemic Index

Food	Glycemic Index (Glucose = 100)	Serving Size (Grams)	Glycemic Load per Serving
Bakery Products and Breads			
Banana cake, made with sugar	47	60	14
Banana cake, made without sugar	55	60	12
Sponge cake, plain	46	63	17
Vanilla cake made from packet mix with vanilla frosting (Betty Crocker)	42	111	24
Apple muffin, made with rolled oats and sugar	44	60	13
Apple muffin, made with rolled oats and without sugar	48	60	9
Waffles, Aunt Jemima	76	35	10
Bagel, white, frozen	72	70	25
Baguette, white, plain	95	30	14
Coarse barley bread, 80% kernels	34	30	7
Hamburger bun	61	30	9

(continued)

Table 2: Glycemic Index (*continued*)

Food	Glycemic Index (Glucose = 100)	Serving Size (Grams)	Glycemic Load per Serving
Kaiser roll	73	30	12
Pumpernickel bread	56	30	7
50% cracked wheat kernel bread	58	30	12
White wheat flour bread, average	75	30	11
Wonder bread, average	73	30	10
Whole wheat bread, average	69	30	9
100% Whole Grain bread (Natural Ovens)	51	30	7
Pita bread, white	68	30	10
Corn tortilla	52	50	12
Wheat tortilla	30	50	8
Beverages			
Coca Cola (US formula)	63	250 mL	16
Fanta, orange soft drink	68	250 mL	23
Lucozade, original (sparkling glucose drink)	95	250 mL	40
Apple juice, unsweetened	41	250 mL	12

(continued)

Cranberry juice cocktail (Ocean Spray)	68	250 mL	24
Gatorade, orange flavor (US formula)	89	250 mL	13
Orange juice, unsweetened, average	50	250 mL	12
Tomato juice, canned, no sugar added	38	250 mL	4
Breakfast Cereals and Related Products			
All-Bran, average	44	30	9
Coco Pops, average	77	30	20
Cornflakes, average	81	30	20
Cream of Wheat	66	250	17
Cream of Wheat, Instant	74	250	22
Grape-Nuts	75	30	16
Muesli, average	56	30	10
Oatmeal, average	55	250	13
Instant oatmeal, average	79	250	21
Puffed wheat cereal	80	30	17
Raisin Bran	61	30	12
Special K (US formula)	69	30	14
Grains			
Pearled barley, average	25	150	11
Sweet corn on the cob	48	60	14

(continued)

Table 2: Glycemic Index (*continued*)

Food	Glycemic Index (Glucose = 100)	Serving Size (Grams)	Glycemic Load per Serving
Couscous	65	150	9
Quinoa	53	150	13
White rice, boiled, type non-specified	72	150	29
Quick cooking white basmati	63	150	26
Brown rice, steamed	50	150	16
Parboiled Converted white rice (Uncle Ben's)	38	150	14
Whole wheat kernels, average	45	50	15
Bulgur, average	47	150	12
Cookies and Crackers			
Graham crackers	74	25	13
Vanilla wafers	77	25	14
Shortbread	64	25	10
Rice cakes, average	82	25	17
Rye crisps, average	64	25	11
Soda crackers	74	25	12
Dairy Products and Alternatives			
Ice cream, regular, average	62	50	8

(continued)

Ice cream, premium (Sara Lee)	38	50	3
Milk, full-fat, average	31	250 mL	4
Milk, skim, average	31	250 mL	4
Reduced-fat yogurt with fruit, average	33	200	11
Fruits			
Apple, average	36	120	5
Banana, raw, average	48	120	11
Dates, dried, average	42	60	18
Grapefruit	25	120	3
Grapes, black	59	120	11
Oranges, raw, average	45	120	5
Peach, average	42	120	5
Peach, canned in light syrup	52	120	9
Pear, raw, average	38	120	4
Pear, canned in pear juice	44	120	5
Prunes, pitted	29	60	10
Raisins	64	60	28
Watermelon	72	120	4

(continued)

Table 2: Glycemic Index (*continued*)

Food	Glycemic Index (Glucose = 100)	Serving Size (Grams)	Glycemic Load per Serving
Beans and Nuts			
Baked beans	40	150	6
Black-eyed peas	50	150	15
Black beans	30	150	7
Chickpeas	10	150	3
Chickpeas, canned in brine	42	150	9
Navy beans, average	39	150	12
Kidney beans, average	34	150	9
Lentils	28	150	5
Soy beans, average	15	150	1
Cashews, salted	22	50	3
Peanuts	13	50	1
Pasta and Noodles			
Fettuccine	32	180	15
Macaroni, average	50	180	24
Macaroni and Cheese (Kraft)	64	180	33
Spaghetti, white, boiled, average	46	180	22

(continued)

Spaghetti, white, boiled 20 min	58	180	26
Spaghetti, whole-grain, boiled	42	180	17
Snack Foods			
Corn chips, plain, salted	42	50	11
Fruit Roll-Ups	99	30	24
M & M's, peanut	33	30	6
Microwave popcorn, plain, average	65	20	7
Potato chips, average	56	50	12
Pretzels, oven-baked	83	30	16
Snickers Bar, average	51	60	18
Vegetables			
Green peas	54	80	4
Carrots, average	39	80	2
Parsnips	52	80	4
Baked russet potato	111	150	33
Boiled white potato, average	82	150	21
Instant mashed potato, average	87	150	17
Sweet potato, average	70	150	22
Yam, average	54	150	20
Miscellaneous			
Hummus (chickpea salad dip)	6	30	0

(continued)

Table 2: Glycemic Index (*continued*)

Food	Glycemic Index (Glucose = 100)	Serving Size (Grams)	Glycemic Load per Serving
Chicken nuggets, frozen, reheated in microwave oven 5 min	46	100	7
Pizza, plain baked dough, served with parmesan cheese and tomato sauce	80	100	22
Pizza, Super Supreme (Pizza Hut)	36	100	9
Honey, average	61	25	12

Source: "Glycemic Index and Glycemic Load for 100+ Foods," *Harvard Health Publications*, August 27, 2015, http://www.health.harvard.edu/ diseases-and-conditions/glycemic_index_and_glycemic_load_for_100 _foods.

Whole Grains

Whole grains are one type of complex carbohydrate that contain vitamins, minerals, fiber, and other nutrients that work together to protect our health. Whole grains are especially high in B vitamins and contain all three parts of the grain: the bran, germ, and endosperm (the part of a seed that acts as a food store for the developing plant embryo, usually containing starch with protein and other nutrients). These take longer to break down, making it easier for your body to regulate (see Table 3).

Table 3: Whole Grains

---

amaranth (ancient grain similar to rice or maize)

barley

brown rice

buckwheat

bulgur (cracked wheat)

kamut (lots of nutrients; rich, buttery flavor)

millet (ancient heart-healthy grain)

oats

quinoa

rye

sorghum (ancient cereal grain)

spelt

teff (colorful fine grain)

wild rice

Gut the Gluten

I've talked a lot about the problem with gluten, which is in many grain products such as wheat, rye, and barley (see Table 4).

It is difficult to digest and can wreak havoc on your system, particularly if you have a leaky gut, celiac disease, or a gluten sensitivity. There are estimates that nearly 1 in 133 Americans suffers from celiac disease, and approximately 1 in 6 has gluten sensitivity. As I explained in previous chapters, gluten can lead to serious illnesses, including

Caveat: Grains can be hard on the digestive system, so it's a good idea to soak them overnight. One way to soak them is to mix in some water with yogurt or lemon juice.

arthritis, autoimmune diseases, chronic fatigue, and even cancer. For more information on gluten, read my *Guide to a Gluten-Free Diet.*

Table 4: Common Grains with Gluten

barley
bulgar
couscous
durum
einkorn
kamut
malt
rye
semolina
spelt
triticale
wheat bran
wheat germ
wheat starch[2]

The Best Vegetables for a Healthy Gut Diet

When it comes to veggies, eating a rainbow of colors will supply your body with important, healthy phytochemicals that can boost your immune system. The more variety, the better. Some of the beneficial nutrients you will consume include flavonoids (antioxidants), carotene, fiber, and phytonutrients. Green is one of the most important colors to have in your healthy gut diet, so pile the leafy greens like spinach, kale, and chard onto your plate for the most nutrient-rich carbohydrates. The darker the leaves, the more nutrients in the vegetable.

Healthy Gut Diet Suggestions and Replacements

It's important to read labels on packages carefully. Here are some things to look for and to avoid:

Suggestion: Avoid white-flour bread, crackers, snacks, and cookies.

Replacement: Choose whole-grain breads (sourdough, sprouted, or 100 percent whole wheat), crackers, and cookies without additives or hydrogenated oils. White flour has been refined and bleached for extra softness and whiteness. The refining process leaves only the endosperm part of the grain and removes the bran, germ, and husk, which are good for you. Whole grains, on the other hand, retain the nutrients found in the original grain because they are milled in their entirety and not refined. Substances such as iron, niacin, thiamin, riboflavin, folate, vitamin B6, magnesium, zinc, and fiber can often be found in whole grains that are intact. Even with added nutrients, white-flour foods are still a poor nutritional choice.

Suggestion: Avoid boxed cereals and pancake mixes.

Replacement: Make oatmeal or homemade pancakes/waffles with whole grains. Boxed cereals and pancake mixes are extremely refined foods and are often full of unnecessary sugars, additives, and flavorings. Many breakfast cereals are highly fortified with hard-to-digest synthetic vitamins and minerals added during processing that were not in the original product. Additionally, cereal processing often involves high heat and high temperatures that can deplete or destroy nutrients (even in cereals sold in health food stores).

Suggestion: Avoid canned fruits and vegetables.

Replacement: Choose fresh (or frozen) fruits and vegetables, especially lots of leafy greens. Buy organic or locally grown whenever possible. Canned fruits and veggies often have syrups, salts, and other additives to make them last for long periods of time on the shelf. Fresh produce offers antioxidants and flavonoids. Buying frozen produce allows you to eat a variety of fruits and vegetables all year round, even when out of season.

Suggestion: Avoid soft drinks and juice concentrates full of sugars and additives.

Replacement: Drink more water to quench your thirst and try adding a bit of lemon, lime, or orange. If you must drink juice, squeeze your own and dilute with water to lessen the sugar concentration (especially important for children).

Sweeteners Equal Sour Stomach

Most people have a sweet tooth, which has been the case since the dawn of time. But sugar or its substitutes, artificial sweeteners, have been the cause of myriad health problems, including diabetes. Americans in particular consume more than 33 percent of the world's sugar, which amounts to ten million tons annually. I will explain why it is important to choose natural sweeteners and how to break your sugar habit.

White Refined Sugar

The most commonly used sweetener is white refined sugar, the kind that is often added to coffee, cookie dough, and cake batter. It is made from either sugarcane or sugar beets that are stripped of vitamins, minerals, and nutrients. Cane stalks are shredded and squeezed to extract their natural juice, which is boiled until it thickens and molasses-rich sugar crystals begin to form. The crystals are sent to a rapidly spinning centrifuge to remove the molasses and leave pure, naturally white sugar crystals. The sugar crystals are then dried. Refined sugar, which is devoid of all nutrients, can stay on the shelf forever.

Sugar Is Made with Cattle Bones

It is a little-known fact that after sugarcane stalks are crushed to separate the juice from the pulp, the juice is processed and heated to crystallize and is then filtered and bleached with bone char from cows, which is what gives it that pristine white color. There are some certified cane sugars that do not use bone char in their processing, such as beet sugar and organic. Make sure to check labels. Organic sugar is either minimally processed or not refined at all. Bone char is not on the National Organic Program's National List of Allowed and Prohibited Substances, so organic sugar cannot contain bone char. In fact, organic sugars are only milled and never go to refineries where bone char filters are used.[3]

Table 5: Refined Sugars

brown sugar
high-fructose corn syrup
powdered sugar
turbinado sugar
white sugar

Why Is Refined Sugar So Bad for Us?

Refined sugar depresses the immune system and can actually make the body deficient of vitamins and minerals. In order to properly digest excess sugar, the body will be required to use its own store of nutrients, particularly B vitamins. Additionally, refined forms of sugar will elevate the body's own blood sugar levels without the balance of healthful nutrients. Consuming large amounts of refined sugar causes blood glucose (sugar) swings in the body that can lead to the development of chronic illnesses, including diabetes, arthritis, and other conditions (see Table 6).

Table 6: Conditions Associated with Refined Sugar

arthritis

asthma

cancer

candida

dental decay

depression

diabetes

headaches

heart disease

hyperactivity

immune system illnesses

infections

kidney disease

liver disease

obesity

osteoporosis[4]

Tips for Breaking Your Sugar Habit

Let's face it. For many of us, sugar is the food equivalent to heroin, and kicking it out of our diet can be extremely difficult. But it *can* be done by making some simple changes to your daily eating habits. Here are six relatively painless ways to cut or reduce your sugar intake:

1. **Watch for hidden sugar.** Sugar is hidden everywhere, especially in packaged foods. Beware of products claiming to be "natural" or "low fat," which are often loaded with sweeteners and sugars designed to get you hooked. Sugar can hide behind a variety of aliases, including fructose, syrup, sucrose, or molasses.

2. **Make it yourself.** Preparing your own meals and snacks lets you determine exactly how much sugar is going into your diet. If you get a craving for something sweet, substitute sugar with other flavors such as vanilla or citrus zest, which gives you the taste without the calories. I realize not everyone has to time to do this, but DIY puts you in the driver's seat when it comes to sugar intake.

3. **Eat bridge snacks during the day.** Eating only three squares a day is not necessarily the best way to avoid reaching for that sweet treat. Having healthful bridge snacks such as nuts or fresh fruit throughout the day will actually keep your blood sugar steady. When you feel hungry during the day, especially when you are busy and need to recharge, you are more likely to want a sugar fix. But empty sugary treats won't keep you feeling full or energized for

long; you will eventually crash and find yourself looking for your next fix.

5. **Trick your brain**. Believe it or not, eating isn't the only way to feel full. When sweet smells are detected by our olfactory receptors, the appetite control centers in our brain will receive a message that the food has been consumed even if you haven't taken a bite. The next time you are craving a sweet treat, try inhaling vanilla extract. I know it sounds strange, but inhaling pure vanilla extract or vanilla essential oil will cut your cravings. You can smell it directly from the bottle or place a few drops on a handkerchief and sniff it throughout the day. Ideally, smell the scent at least three times a day for thirty seconds each time, but more is also OK.[5]

6. **Cut back gradually**. For some, going cold turkey on sugar is darn near impossible. If this is the case for you, gradually wean yourself off, which will train your body to naturally lower its desire for sugary fixes. If you are used to adding three teaspoons of sugar to your coffee, for example, cut back to two for a week, then one, and finally none. I promise that your body and taste buds will eventually readjust, and you will actually prefer unsweetened beverages.

Everyone is different, so the amount of time it takes to make these changes depends on the individual and willpower. But if you commit yourself to making these changes, you will be able to see the progress fairly quickly.

Artificial Sugar Is Not a Healthy Alternative
You've already read about some of the dangers of artificial sugar, which can actually cause obesity, and neurological and immune system disorders. The most common artificial sweeteners are aspartame (AminoSweet, NutraSweet, Equal, Spoonful, and Equal-Measure), saccharin (Sweet'N Low), and sucralose (Splenda), a newer sweetener that can lead to thyroid and other hormonal problems. There are usually pink or blue packets of these sugar substitutes on restaurant tables. (See Table 7 for natural alternatives to refined sugar.)

Table 7: Natural Sweeteners

---

agave nectar (extracted from core of the Agave plant)

fruit (bananas, berries)

honey (raw)

maple sugar (dehydrated maple syrup)

maple syrup (good source of manganese, zinc, and other nutrients)

molasses (blackstrap molasses is a wonderful source of iron, calcium, copper, potassium, and magnesium)

rapadura (unrefined and unbleached whole cane sugar)

stevia (herb that comes in powder extract or liquid concentrate)

sucanat (does not have the molasses removed, so it retains nutrient value)

xylitol (a low-glycemic sweetener that's safe for diabetics and hypoglycemics)

Fats and Oils

What Is Fat?

There are four general categories of fat: polyunsaturated, monounsaturated, saturated, and trans. With the exception of trans fat, your body needs them all. Fat has gotten a really bad rap, but it contains more energy than both protein and carbs, and it's essential for forming cell membranes and for hormone production. Not getting enough fat can lead to vitamin deficiency because it acts as a carrier for soluble vitamins, including A, D, E, and K. Fat is found in both animal and vegetable products and adds flavor to food in addition to satisfying our hunger.

Good and Bad Fats

Just like carbohydrates and cholesterol, there are good fats and there are bad ones. Good fats are those that have not been hydrogenated (the unhealthy process that turns vegetable oil into margarine) and can be in the form of saturated, monounsaturated, and polyunsaturated fats. Bad fats provide no nutrition for the body and also cause the immune system to malfunction. Good fats, on the other hand (such as saturated fats), are necessary for proper brain function (it is the major fat in the brain), provide important nutrition, and strengthen our cell walls (see Tables 8 and 9).

Table 8: Bad Fats

partially hydrogenated vegetable oils
processed vegetable oils (e.g., soy, canola, corn, cottonseed)
trans fats (should be avoided—period)

Table 9: Good Fats

Healthy Foods with Significant Amounts of Saturated Fats
coconut oil
cultured dairy (i.e., yogurt, kefir, organic butter)
organic, free-range red meat
Healthy Foods with Sources of Monounsaturated Fat
avocado
almonds
canola oil
cashews
hazelnuts
macadamias
olive oil
peanuts
pecans
pistachios
Sources of Polyunsaturated Oils
omega-3 fatty acids
Cold-water fish oils (mackerel, salmon, albacore, tuna, sardines, lake trout)
flax seeds
flaxseed oil
pumpkin seeds
walnuts

Certain polyunsaturated fats (e.g., vegetable oils such as soy, corn, canola, and cottonseed) are overused and contain high amounts of omega-6 fatty acids without the balancing effects of omega-3s and have been shown to depress the immune system over time. Additionally, many of these oils contain harmful free radicals due to the high heat and pressure of the refining process.

How to Purchase Healthy Oils

1. The container must be shielded from light, as light damages healthy oils. Do not buy oils in a clear container.
2. There should be an expiration date on the container. Nutrients have a shelf life. If there are no nutrients in the oil, it can last forever.
3. There should be no high-temperature processing or hydrogenation of the oils, as these destroy the valuable nutrients and create toxins. (Look for expeller or cold-pressed oils found mostly at health-food stores.)

Protein

Proteins, the building blocks of the body, are made up of amino acid chains. They are elements of every cell and necessary for building and repairing tissues. Proteins are also required for healthy muscles, skin, and organs; the nervous system; and proper enzyme function. The immune system uses specialized proteins called antibodies to fight infections. My experience has shown that a lack of protein in the diet will lead to a variety of medical problems, including a poorly functioning immune system and hormonal imbalances.

Where to Get Protein

Protein is in both animal and plant products. However, animal protein is the only source of essential amino acids, which plant products do not contain (see Table 10).

Table 10: Sources of Protein

Animals	Plants
Cheese	Beans
Eggs	Cereal
Fish	Corn
Meat	Legumes
Milk	Rice
Soy	

The Soy Deception

Soy is often touted in the media as a good source of protein, but this couldn't be further from the truth. Soy is presently the cheapest crop to grow in the United States, and because it is widely available, it is promoted as a healthy food. Soy contains enzyme inhibitors that block the absorption of essential minerals, including calcium, magnesium, zinc, manganese, and iron. If that's not bad enough, large amounts of refined soy can cause deficiencies in vitamins B12, D, E, and K. Fermented forms of soy (e.g., miso, natto, and tempeh) are much healthier than those in soy milk, cheese, yogurt, hot dogs, and burgers. Vegetarians beware: soy should not be the major source of protein in your diet. I would go as far as to say eliminate all refined soy products from your diet completely. For more about soy, see my book *The Soy Deception*.

Red Meat

Red meat can be a good source of protein if the animals are grass fed or wild game—not from factory farms. The best source of red meat is organic, which is free of antibiotics and hormones. Although frequently vilified in the press, red meat contains the full complement of B vitamins and amino acids and has easily absorbable minerals.

Poultry

Poultry such as chicken and turkey can be a healthy source of protein if it is from an organic, free-range farm that gives the fowl room to roam, natural sunlight, and a natural diet. Look for poultry raised by farmers who do not use feed treated with pesticides or give their stock antibiotics and/or growth hormones. Poultry from a good source is full of essential amino acids and is high in tryptophan.

The Chicken or the Egg?

If I were to choose, I'd say the egg, which is a perfect food. The egg contains the full complement of amino acids and large amounts of the essential nutrients choline (important for liver function, brain development, nerve function, muscle movement, and maintaining a healthy metabolism) and lutein (good for the eyes). The same caveats for the poultry apply here. Free range, organic, certified humane only.

Beans and Lentils

Although not complete proteins because they are missing some of the essential amino acids, beans and lentils are still a good source of protein, especially when paired with rice. Beans and lentils should be cleaned, rinsed, and soaked prior to cooking to loosen skins, ease digestion, and minimize the cooking time and the gassiness they often produce. Another plus is that they are inexpensive and extremely versatile, while providing nutrients such as iron, zinc, potassium, magnesium, manganese, phosphorus, and thiamin.

Fish

Fish is high in protein as well as a good source of vitamins and minerals. It contains omega-3 fatty acids that are linked to improved blood flow, increased growth of brain cells, improved mood, and lower rates of depression. Good choices include cold-water fatty fish such as salmon, bluefish, herring, sardines, mackerel, tuna, and trout. Wild caught is best (avoid farm-raised fish, as they have toxic items such as dyes and polychlorinated biphenyls [PCBs] from the feed they are given and also have an altered fatty acid profile compared to wild-caught fish). Protein derived from fish oils is also great for the heart, eyes, skin, hair, and nails.

> **Caveat**: Beware of fish that swim in polluted waters. Two of the most common pollutants in the fish are PCBs and mercury, which can build up in the body over time. It's important to avoid fish with high levels of these toxic elements. People who are especially at risk to toxins are young children and pregnant women.

Nuts and Seeds

Nuts and seeds are some of the healthiest foods on the planet. They

Caveat: Avoid nuts with partially hydrogenated oils (e.g., soybean oil), which are an unnecessary source of harmful trans fat and have no nutritional value.

grow from plants and trees and are full of vitamins, minerals, antioxidants, phytochemicals, and phytosterols (a.k.a. plant sterols, which are a family of molecules found in the cell membranes of plants). Nuts are a good source of healthy fats that help build healthy immune and nervous systems. Although high in calories, the nutrients in nuts provide the body with an excellent source of protein and energy (see Table 11).

Table 11: Nutritious Nuts and Seeds

almonds

Brazil nuts

cashews

hazelnuts

pecans

pumpkin seeds

Roast Your Own Nuts

1. Soak raw nuts overnight in large bowl with 2–3 teaspoons of Celtic sea salt and water (add more or less salt to taste).
2. Strain the saltwater.
3. Arrange nuts on cookie sheet and place in oven. Cook at 150–175°F overnight or until dry.

Go Nuts

Nuts and seeds are best when bought raw (preferably organic) in packages, not in bulk bins where they might not be fresh. Here are more buying tips:

- Avoid commercially packaged nut mixes that have salt, flavorings, and processed vegetable oils. Buy fresh raw nuts, preferably in packages, and make your own mixes.
- Steer clear of roasted and salted nuts sold in grocery stores.

Salt

Another food "addiction" that grips many Americans (second only to refined sugar) is refined salt, which is found in most processed products. Table salt, which is refined white salt that is very fine, is in nearly 100 percent sodium chloride and contains additives such as iodine—added to prevent goiter. What is not well known is that refined table salt also contains sugar and aluminum. The sugar is used stabilize the iodine and as an anticaking agent. Avoid table salt, as it has little nutritional value.

Unrefined Salt

Unrefined salt, such as Celtic sea salt, is the only kind that retains its nutritional content and preserves the vital balance of ocean minerals. It contains more than eighty minerals that the body needs to function at its best (see Table 12).

Table 12: Benefits of Unrefined Salt

balances blood sugar

helps relax the body for sleep

improves brain function

prevents muscle cramps

prevents varicose veins

prevents osteoporosis

raises pH in the body

regulates blood pressure (if hydrated)

thins mucous

Go Paleo

Finally, the answer to "What kind of *diet* should I be on?" is Paleo. Popularized in a book by author Robb Wolf, it is based on the Paleolithic food groups eaten by our hunter/gatherer ancestors. The Paleo diet consists of lean proteins that support strong muscles, healthy bones, and optimal immune function; fruits and vegetables; and healthy fats from nuts and seeds, avocados, olive oil, fish oil, and grass-fed meats. It also involves drinking lots of water and eliminating refined food, dairy, and starches.

In my estimation, it is the healthiest diet, especially for a leaky gut, as well as the most satisfying. Research shows that our modern diet—full of refined foods, trans fats, and sugar (everything you've read about in this chapter and book)—is at the at the root of diseases such as obesity, diabetes, heart disease, autoimmune disorders, Alzheimer's, depression, and cancer. Eating a Paleo diet, combined with correcting nutritional and hormonal imbalances with a program designed by your holistic doctor, and adopting a healthy lifestyle has worked for a vast majority of my patients suffering from leaky gut and its resulting illnesses and conditions.

Healthy Eating Starts Today!

I hope this book has helped you, or someone you love, who is suffering from conditions that we now know are rooted in leaky gut syndrome (LGS). My medical training and two decades as a holistic physician has led me to conclude, like Hippocrates, that all disease starts with the gut. Since Hippocrates's time, thousands of scientific studies have been conducted on LGS, and an increasing number of traditional doctors are also seeing the light at the end of the gastrointestinal tunnel.

Remember, there are no medications that treat the underlying cause of irritable bowel syndrome (IBS), Crohn's disease, ulcerative colitis, and many other illnesses. Why not? Because treating most gut problems can be successfully accomplished through natural therapies that Big Pharma cannot patent. Without patents, the pharmaceutical industry has no way to profit. No profit, no interest—it's that simple. So it's up the pioneers in the holistic field to educate patients about how to treat their GI issues, which include cleaning up their diet and identifying and removing food allergies. None of these treatments and therapies I recommend will put you in debt, but they might just change your life for the better.

Now that you understand how your gut works, what can go wrong, and how to correct it, you have the tools you need to be healthier and, hopefully, disease-free for as long as possible. If your doctor doesn't suggest the tests I recommended in Chapter 1, which I believe should be standard operating procedure for any checkup, it is time for you to find another doctor who is willing work with you. I can't emphasize enough how important it is to get the right tests done so that your doctor can evaluate your body's nutritional status, including deficiencies that cause inflammation, IBS, asthma, acne, headaches, fatigue, autoimmune diseases, depression, and myriad conditions described in this book.

Finally, if you take away only one piece of advice, let it be this: start eating a healthy diet *today*! Sure, I can correct vitamin and mineral deficiencies with supplements, but you can (and should) be an active participant in your own treatment by giving your body (and your gut) the nutrients it needs to function optimally. Leaky gut occurs, in large part, from eating a poor diet, and it can be cured. It's worked for me, for members of my family, and for the patients whose stories you have just read.

I've provided you with a common-sense approach to LGS that includes natural, nontoxic therapies; what to eat; what to cut out; and how to drink enough water for your weight, which will supply you with the nutrients you need to heal your leaky gut. The human body is designed perfectly if we treat it well. Please cherish and nourish yours.

Again, I encourage you to visit my website and blog at http://www.drbrownstein.com, where you can learn more about this and other health issues as well was ask me questions. You can also subscribe to my *Natural Way to Health* newsletter for the latest news on medical discoveries and holistic treatment (naturalway@newsmax.com).

To all our health,

DB

Notes

Introduction

1 "U.S. Food & Drug Administration," US Department of Health & Human Services, accessed April 13, 2007, https://www.fda.gov/drugs/developmentapprovalprocess/developmentresources/druginteractionslabeling/ucm110632.htm.

Chapter 1

1 "Stool Analysis," *WebMD*, http://www.webmd.com/digestive-disorders/stool-analysis#1.

2 "Upper Gastrointestinal (UGI) Series," *WebMD*, http://www.webmd.com/digestive-disorders/upper-gastrointestinal-ugi-series#1.

3 Norma Devault, "What Is the Difference Between Good Bacteria & Bad Bacteria," *Livestrong*, September 26, 2015, http://www.livestrong.com/article/337181-what-is-the-difference-between-good-bacteria-bad-bacteria/.

4 Ibid.

5 "Gut Microbiata for Health," *Healthline*, accessed April 13, 2017, http://www.gutmicrobiataforhealth.com.

Chapter 2

1 "Diseases and Conditions: GERD," *MayoClinic*, January 31, 2014, http://www.mayoclinic.org/diseases-conditions/gerd/basics/symptoms/con-20025201.

2 College of Family Physicians of Canada, "Heartburn: Hints on Dealing with the Discomfort," *Resources*, 2007, http://www.cfpc.ca/projectassets/templates/resource.aspx?id=1382&langType=4105; "Gastroesophageal Reflux Disease and Heartburn," *University of Maryland Medical Center*, http://www.umm.edu/health/medical/reports/articles/gastroesophageal-reflux-disease-and-heartburn; "Heartburn or Gastroesophageal Reflux Disease," *American College of Gastroenterology*, http://s3.gi.org/patients/cgp/pdf/Wgerd.pdf; "GERD or Acid Reflux or Heartburn," *Cleveland Clinic*, https://my.clevelandclinic.org/health/articles/gastroesophogeal-reflux-disease-gerd; "Heartburn, Gastroesophageal Reflux (GERD), and Gastroesophageal Reflux Disease," *National Digestive Diseases Information Clearinghouse*, https://www.guideline.gov/syntheses/synthesis/50025.

3 "Definition & Facts for Irritable Bowel Syndrome," *National Institute of Diabetes and Digestive and Kidney Diseases*, February 2017, https://www.niddk.nih.gov/health-information/digestive-diseases/irritable-bowel-syndrome.

4 Joe Bowman and Erica Cirino, "The 6 Most Effective Diarrhea Remedies," *Healthline*, accessed August 16, 2016, http://www.healthline.com/health/digestive-health/most-effective-diarrhea-remedies#2.

5 Brett Lashner, "You Won't Believe How This Works: Fecal Transplant; Healthy Gut Flora Defeat Clostridium Difficile Infection," May 30, 2014, https://health.clevelandclinic .org/2014/05/despite-the-ick-factor-fecal-procedure-works -wonders/.

6 NIH US National Library of Medicine, "Mucolipidosis Type IV," *Genetics Home Reference*, accessed January 13, 2017, https://ghr.nlm.nih.gov/condition/mucolipidosis-type -iv.

7 https://medlineplus.gov.

8 Fu Huwez, "Mastic Gum Kills *H. pylori*," *NEJM* 339, no. 26 (December 24, 1998); M. Odashima, "Induction of a 72-kDa Heat-Shock Protein in Cultured Rat Gastric Mucosal Cells and Rat Gastric Mucosa by Zinc L-Carnosine," *Dig. Dis. Sci.* 47, no. 12 (December 2002): 2799–2804; T. Matsukura, "Applicability of Zinc Complex of L-Carnosine for Medical Use," *Biochemistry* 65, no. 7 (July 2000): 817–23.

9 http://www.ncbi.nlm.nih.gov/pubmed/23220194.

10 http://www.atmjournal.org/article/view/6371/7502; https://www .ncbi.nlm.nih.gov/pubmed/19879118.

11 http://www.mayoclinic.org/diseases-conditions/peptic-ulcer/ basics/lifestyle-home-remedies/con-20028643.

Chapter 3

1 David Brownstein, *Overcoming Arthritis* (West Bloomfield, MI: Medical Alternative Press, 2001).

2 http://blog.arthritis.org/living-with-arthritis/fibromyalgia -diet/#more-553.

3 Marie Pasinski with Jodie Gould, *Beautiful Brain, Beautiful You* (New York, NY; Hyperion, 2011).

4 http://www.webmd.com/osteoporosis/guide/understanding -osteoporosis-symptoms.

5 http://www.cdc.gov/cfs/causes/risk-groups.html.

6 https://well.blogs.nytimes.com/2016/07/07/gut-bacteria
-are-different-in-people-with-chronic-fatigue-syndrome/
https://microbiomejournal.biomedcentral.com/articles/10
.1186/s401.

7 Jodie Gould, *HIGH: Six Principles for Guilt-Free Pleasure and Escape* (Center City, MI; Hazelden, 2015).

Chapter 4

1 Amy Myers and David Brownstein, *The Autoimmune Solution.*

2 http://www.jdrf.com.

3 "Duodenal Mucosa of Patients with Type 1 Diabetes Shows Distinctive Inflammatory Profile and Microbiota," https://academic.oup.com/jcem/article-lookup/doi/10.1210/jc.2016-3222 (forthcoming).

4 Excerpted from David Brownstein, *Drugs That Don't Work and Natural Therapies That Do!* (West Bloomfield, MI: Medical Alternative Press), 75–99.

5 http://www.lupus.org.

6 http://www.furtherfood.com.

7 Jeri Burtchell, "Leaky Gut Syndrome Implicated in Multiple Sclerosis," *Healthline*, September 25, 2014, http://www.healthline.com/health-news/leaky-gut-implicated-in-multiple-sclerosis-092514.

8 David Brownstein, *Overcoming Thyroid Disorders* (West Bloomfield, MI: Medical Alternative Press, 2008), 100.

9 Ibid.

Chapter 5

1 http://www.foodallergy.org.

2 David Brownstein, *Drugs That Don't Work and Natural Therapies That Do!* (West Bloomfield, MI: Medical Alternative Press, 2009)

3 http://www.healthline.com/health/anaphylactic-shock.

4 Association for Comprehensive NeuroTherapy, "Seed, Feed and Weed to Reverse Inflammatory Disease," *Latitudes* (online newsletter), http://latitudes.org/seed-feed-weed-reverse-inflammatory-disease/.

5 Doris Day with Jodie Gould, *Beyond Beauty* (New York: Center Street Press, forthcoming 2018).

6 Ibid.

7 Julien Farel, phone interview with NYC salon owner and manufacturer of hair products, October 2016.

8 Robynne Chutkan, *Gutbliss* (New York: Avery, 2014)

Chapter 6

1 www.hopkinsmedicine.org/health/healthy_aging/healthy_body/the-brain-gut-connection.

2 http://naturalnews.com/2017-01-28-new-study-finds-how-microorganisms-living-in-thehuman-gut-could-affect-your-physiology.html.

3 D. D. Burns, *Feeling Good: The New Mood Therapy* (New York: Avon, 1999); R. L. Leahy and S. J. Holland, *Treatment Plans and Interventions for Depression and Anxiety Disorders* (New York: Guilford Press, 2000).

4 David Brownstein, *Dr. David Brownstein's Natural Way to Health* (Newsmax newsletter) 4, no. 12 (December 2011): 3–5.

5 "Prozac Drug Information," *Prescribers Digital Reference*, accessed February 2017, http://www.pdr.net/drug-summary/Prozac-fluoxetine-hydrochloride-3205.2826.

6 Jodie Gould, *HIGH: Six Principles for Guilt-Free Pleasure and Escape* (Center City, MI: Hazelden, 2015).

7 http://www.thelancet.com/journals/lancet/article/PIIS0140
-6736%2810%2962227-1/abstract.

8 http://www.ncbi.nlm.nih.gov/pubmed/20034331; http://www.live
beaming.com/2013/04/food-intolerance-adhd/; http://www.ncbi
.nlm.nih.gov/pubmed/9368236; http://www.ncbi.nlm.nih.gov/pu
bmed/9368235; http://www.thelancet.com/journals/lancet/articl
e/PIIS0140-6736%2810%2962227-1/abstract.

9 Marie Pasinski with Jodie Gould, *Beautiful Brain, Beautiful You* (New York: Hyperion, 2011).

10 https://medicalxpress.com; http://www.naturalnews.com.

11 http://www.alz.org/dementia/types-of-dementia.asp.

12 http://www.jama.ama-assn.org/cgi/content/full/304/17/1903.

13 http://www.naturalnews.com.

14 Tim Buie, "Gastrointestinal Problems in Autism and the Brain-Gut Connection," *Quantum University*, November 19, 2016, https://iquim.org/dr-buie/fullvideo/.

Chapter 7

1 http://www.npr.org/sections/thesalt/2013/07/09/200465360/
the-science-of-twinkies-how-do-they-last-so-long.

2 David Brownstein and Sheryl Shenefelt, *The Guide to Healthy Eating* (Birmingham, MI: Healthy Living, 2010).

3 http://www.huffingtonpost.com/2015/01/05/sugar-vegan-bone
-char-yikes_n_6391496.html; Vegetarian Resource Group, http://
www.vrg.org/journal/vj2007issue4/2007_issue4_sugar.php.

4 David Brownstein and Sheryl Shenefelt, *The Guide to Healthy Eating* (Birmingham, MI: Healthy Living, 2010).

5 http://www.care2.com/greenliving/the-scent-that-stop-cra
vings-in-their-tracks.html.

Index

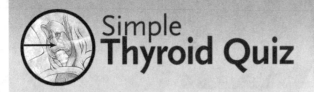 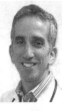

Simple
Thyroid Quiz

Is Your Thyroid Secretly Hurting You?
Find Out in Minutes . . .

Have you recently been feeling 'not quite right'? Do you struggle with losing weight or have unexplained fatigue or brain fog? The answer could be your thyroid! **Take this online quiz to find out.**

Thyroid disorders have now been linked to 59 major diseases including **heart disease**, **arthritis**, **obesity**, **chronic fatigue**, **diabetes**, and more. Your thyroid is a small, butterfly-shaped gland in your neck, weighing only about 1 ½ ounces. And while it may be small in size, many health experts consider your thyroid to be a master gland when it comes to controlling your body.

Dr. David Brownstein, one of the nation's leading experts on natural thyroid health, has created his own thyroid health quiz. It allows you to easily assess your thyroid health risk in just a matter of minutes.

Test Your Thyroid Health Today!

SimpleThyroidTest.com/Gut

Powered by newsmax health

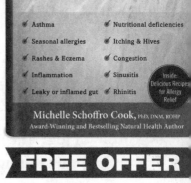